Psycho-Spiritual Healing AFTER An Abortion

Douglas R. Crawford
and
Michael T. Mannion

Sheed & Ward

All Scripture citations taken from the New American Bible.

Sheed & Ward™ is a service of National Catholic Reporter Publishing Company, Inc.

Library of Congress Catalog Card Number: 88-63847

ISBN: 1-55612-246-2

Published by: Sheed & Ward
                115 E. Armour Blvd. P.O. Box 419492
                Kansas City, MO 64141

To order, call: (800) 333-7373

Contents

Dedication

This book is dedicated to the
women who trusted us on
their journeys to
rediscover
themselves and their God.

Acknowledgements

Special thanks to Sue, Heather, and Michele for their love and support.

We offer a very special word of thanks to Beverly Gatti who patiently and proficiently typed the manuscript for this book.

—For those of psychology and faith—
—For the counselor and clergy person—
who wish to work together in
helping one heal
AFTER
an abortion

1.

Introduction

Like all matters of human suffering, the causes of pain and the path to healing can be viewed in a variety of ways. Every point of view about the origins of suffering has purpose and meaning and can evoke argument or agreement, confusion or understanding. The understanding of the why and wherefore of pain may not require agreement or disagreement by one who sees it. It might be approached without any bias whatsoever for that matter. Our purpose in this book is to relate to you, the reader, our experience of three representative women who have each had an abortion and have each sought to ease their aftermath distress by reaching out to two other people: one, a psychologist and one, a priest—individuals who have tried to be present to them in a healing way.

From the viewpoint of a psychologist or clergyperson, the distress of each woman may be regarded at first as a pain exhibiting stated and/or observable symptoms that limit everyday functions or well-being. This psychological point of view, however, may not take into account what meaning the abortion had and will have in the future for the woman, her family and friends, and her relationship with God. The focus is rather on the diagnosis and treatment plan and how that

1

might help her function personally and relationally in healthy ways.

From the viewpoint of the priest, the distress and pain of each woman may be regarded at first as a pain deeply rooted in her decision to abort her unborn child. In doing so, she not only denied her child's life, but denied a part of herself and rejected the gift of God's life in her. The focus is on her journey to wholeness through a personal experience of God's love and forgiveness.

Neither view should be seen in isolation or in opposition to the other. The psychological and the spiritual can and do complement one another. In our counseling, our personal approaches have often found complement and completion in the other. Whenever a psychological method is employed, the hope is for a positive spiritual outcome. When a psychological term is defined, a faith perspective is sought. Good psychology lends itself to good spirituality.

In our work together, we attempt to speak a blended language that transcends and unifies our counseling goals. Out of this effort came the idea of this book. A book that hopefully will help you, the reader, to work towards understanding the whole process of healing a person who hurts.

For those of you who read this book with the intention of counseling a woman who has had an abortion, please understand that both the psychological and the spiritual aspects presuppose people of faith. Counseling by a psychologist is inadequate and incomplete without recognition of her faith dimension and struggle. The counselor who supports her with this recognition can then expect the woman's healing process to be fruitful. When a clergy person is simply added to the process as a polite afterthought, the process will not be whole. At the same time, it is inadequate for a clergyperson to expect God to "do it all" without recognizing the need for psychological counseling skills. The grace that builds on nature is the grace that works through nature. This grace is God's personal invitation to the woman—an invitation to accept his loving embrace and thus be healed.

Faith is not the icing on the cake. It is integrative to the whole healing journey that takes into account the fact that we experience the depth of our spirituality through the fullness of our humanity and that we are most free when we choose to give life—with all its implications and consequences. This book is a statement that the spiritual and psychological not only can complement each other, but must do so--for the welfare of the woman who seeks to be whole, for the memory of the child who cried out to be born.

"I came that they might have life and have it to the full." (John 10:10)

2.

Three Women:
From Brokenness
to Healing

When a psychologist, priest or counselor assumes the responsibility of being a helper, there may at first be a strong desire to seek therapeutic success vis-a-vis set goals and methods that reportedly have a high probability of returning the woman to a state of greater health. Our desire for success and fulfillment as helpers may lead us to choose and believe in certain methods and techniques. Even though the woman is influenced through our experience as counselors, we by no means are in isolation in our effort to bring about her greater health. We must seek the give-and-take of sharing the woman's experience combined with our insights. This is a sharing that will give rise to understanding between the woman and ourselves, the woman and the child, and the child and the woman and God. Knowledge is the objective fact we communicate. Insight is a product of her reflection about her own life. We feed back to the woman what she has taught us about herself.

As a result, the give and take of the woman's experience and our goals need to be whole and consist of a synthesis that is flexible and open-ended. The reader is encouraged to view each representative woman described below and the therapeutic goals as a map—not the actual territory of the helping process—that is, an experience ever-changing each time we sit, listen and talk. Thus, the counselor must be open to recognize always that only the woman can teach us who she is. We must not let our preconceived strategies, stereotypes and judgments stand in the way of her discovery of who she is. When this occurs, the counselor is truly a helper.

Helen

Helen, age 21, was a heart-centered type of person who often found herself driven to achieve and would rarely stumble in her efforts. Her parents expected much. So did she, of herself. She felt if she failed, she would be less of a person and consequently had difficulty admitting she was wrong. Sometimes she was confused as to how she might please her mother, something very important to her. On the one hand, she was encouraged to try new things and explore new lands. On the other hand, she was ever-reminded not to make mistakes. Thus, she feared failing and protected herself vigorously. Overwhelmed by over-seeking of the right kind of effort, she found herself frequently either seeking respect or over-thinking and second-guessing almost everything. It seemed that she hardly ever trusted the rightness of her own decisions, often seeking to please everyone and feeling somewhat fulfilled when she walked the tightrope of keeping everybody happy—her special fulfillment in life.

In her effort to show a good appearance to self and others, she tried to project herself as subtle, self-assured and dogmatic. She constantly sought to give to others in an effort to prove to herself that she was worth something and was someone. She hardly ever said exactly what she felt—that was too dangerous and might cost her rejection. A price too dear to pay. It was easier to tell people what they wanted to hear (as best she understood that) and then at least maintain some level of intimacy and friendship.

Helen's basic temperament was centered upon trying to understand the meaning of her feelings since she was quite concerned with how she felt and why. She worked as a teacher and was often willing to share inspirations and idealisms and see the best in her students, especially when they or she succeeded in her goals. This was not unlike how her parents related to her.

Helen could help others understand how they felt and why, experience empathy, arouse curiosity, supply new possibilities, tackle problems and prepare for the future. At the same time, she needed others to help her apply practical solutions to difficult problems, be mindful of details and facts and show patience.

Theresa

Theresa, a woman of 35, expressed to almost everyone a need to be loyal and very rarely deviated from conventional thought. Theresa was the first-born of five children and was frequently entrusted with many responsibilities in the family. She learned at an early age that everything has a place. She found her self-worth in doing the right thing, the right way, at the right time. She always dressed well, her room was neat, her life was neat. Everything had to fit in. She was secure in a world that was totally organized. She perceived herself in control and with power as long as the world was organized. A change in schedule or plans, especially at the last minute, produced intense anxiety. Flexibility was often impossible because it meant instability.

In her effort to sort out apprehensions about tomorrow which might bring about unpredictable and unplanned-for events, she was often rigid in pursuing her goals of success. With the ensuing anxiety, she could be dominating, unrealistic and fault-finding when pressed to accept the spontaneous in life.

Theresa's basic temperament was centered upon acquiring knowledge, and she was quite concerned with predicting and controlling the environment—again another symbol of seeking security. She worked in computer sciences and seemed to be constantly thinking, planning and synthesizing ideas. Her world was well-ordered and a comfortable place to be.

Theresa could help others understand and analyze the world about them and see the relationship of the chain of events in themselves, be they fortunate or unfortunate. At the same time, she needed others to help her understand the feelings of others instead of just how they thought; to help her find reconciliation as well as justice, and to see the difficulties that come from looking at the world and people from only a logical point of view minus compassion and a sense of enjoying life's pleasures. She seemed to feel she did not have the right to enjoy life unless she first figured it out.

Ingrid

Ingrid, aged 17, was quite set in her ways and was used to getting her way most of the time. Her parents needed her to accept them. She learned this instinctively at an early age and knew how to play them off against one another. She routinely avoided any behavior construed as weakness in her life. She wasn't afraid of asserting herself in most situations. Ensnared by over-seeking attention and recognition, she frequently found herself craving an environment of peer support where her domination would be recognized and vengeance displayed. She could be arrogant in her sense of justly demanding what she needed.

In her effort to be in control, she would at times betray long-standing friendships and loyalties, withhold feelings of tenderness and gentleness, and show few signs of weakness.

Ingrid's basic temperament was centered upon plotting and planning to whatever extent needed to get what she wanted. Her wants were usually based upon short-range emotional gains rather than any resemblance to long-range goals.

Ingrid was known as a good listener and could help others to focus their efforts and set priorities. At the same time, it would be difficult for her to help others plan for their future since she could not plan for her own. She needed others to help her prepare for unforeseen problems, incorporate new information and see beyond the present. Her motto was, "if it feels good, do it."

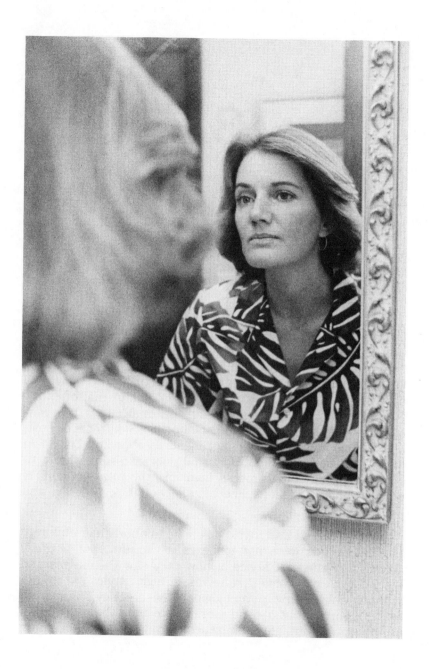

3.

Understanding the Pain

In the preceding chapter, we portrayed a few of the essential features of the representative women with whom we have worked. Later, in Chapter 4 (The Counseling and Healing Process: A Holistic Approach), we'll outline how each woman was helped in the counseling process. In this chapter, we will describe the psychological and spiritual fallout that often occurs after an abortion—a painful aftermath that has now commonly come to be called Post-Abortion Syndrome or Post-Traumatic Stress Disorder as related to abortion. This pain calls for a therapeutic and spiritual response—one which encompasses a healing process involving the total personality in a woman's Actions, Feelings, Thoughts, Energy and Relationships.

Helen, Theresa and Ingrid all chose to abort their children. Their decisions were not made in a vacuum, but actually grew out of the past styles of how they saw themselves and how they expressed themselves. These styles were not pathological in any psychological sense. They, like other women, sought out a counselor, not to help them deal with an abortion, but to seek relief from a myriad of other problems, fears and anxieties, only later in the counseling process revealed as symptomatic of an underlying abortion experience. Their self-image has been traumatized by severe distress. At the core of their damaged self-image is the continued thought that harm has occurred, though they might not have given themselves permission to face that thought, let alone believe they can face and cope with it. They doubt themselves and questions of personal responsibility arise which only accentuate thoughts of guilt. They experience an anxiety that leads to intensified grief, particularly because, in many cases, the cause of the grief has not been faced. Consistent with the writing of Dr. Vincent Rue, of the Sir Thomas More Clinics in California, "A Description of Post-Abortion Syndrome, Diagnostic Criteria," developed from the *Diagnostic And Statistical Manual of Mental Disorders* (widely used in the psychiatric and psychological community), the women we have seen show a variety of overwhelming post-abortion effects.

First, for example, they may re-experience abortion trauma by recalling the actual experience: time of day, place, smells, furniture in the room, mannerisms and personalities of the abortion staff, etc. They may have horrifying dreams of the abortion procedure as well as haunting fantasies about the child. There may be a sense of reliving the experience in action and feeling with possible illusions, hallucinations and flashbacks. The women seem to live with a distress-pending relapse mentality—a fear that it will happen again. At times this fear can possibly be intensified by the presence of pregnant mothers, physicians, hospitals or clinics. These factors may become life-long reminders. There may also be anniversary reactions with significant sadness and bereavement. Unknowingly, at times, women will experience changes in their actions, feelings and thoughts on or about the date of their abortion. The astute counselor may link the change with that date.

Second, there can be persistent avoidance or numbing response to involvement with life after the abortion. There is an avoidance of actions, feelings, thoughts, information, situations, activities and relationships associated with the abortion. The parent or girl friend who thought herself to be helpful by helping to pay for the abortion or even by going with the woman to the abortion clinic might later be very confused and perplexed when the woman rejects her: "I stood by her during the abortion. Why is she rejecting me?" The woman herself may look on the experience and her friend with great disappointment and anger: "Why didn't they speak up and have the courage to tell me I was going to kill my baby?"

An inability to recall the details of the abortion may occur with the hope of "less memory—less pain."

A denial type of lifestyle brings about feelings of detachment and acts of withdrawal, reduced communication and restricted emotions. The woman may have little or no motivation to participate in meaningful relationships; after all, now she knows "it will only lead to another disaster." Sometimes the denial has to do with depression, sometimes revenge, sometimes bitterness. The suppressed (conscious) pain and the repressed (unconscious) pain harden the denial. The pain not faced becomes intensified and energy draining for many other areas of life. The effort to keep the mask of denial in place may result in a drained person left with the haunting question, "Why doesn't anything ever go right in my life?" A woman may seem frozen in time and say such things as, "I haven't changed or grown since my abortion, I feel stagnant." She may have a pessimistic view of the future and seem to perpetuate hopelessness by not expecting a happy life, healthy children and satisfying relationships. Moreover, she may feel she doesn't deserve them.

Third, the ongoing symptoms associated with, but perhaps not initially recognized by the woman may include acts of irritability, hyper-vigilance (always being on guard and defensive), alcohol or substance abuse. There may be expressed anger, guilt or depression. Thoughts of suicide, self-devaluation, difficulty in self-forgiveness, intrusive or non-controllable recollections of the abortion, or difficulty in concentrating may be present. There may also be problems with increased physical energy, falling and staying asleep, or physiological reactivity upon exposure to events or situations that resemble or symbolize an aspect of the trauma. These could well include, for example, sweating, breathing difficulty, tight stomach, nervousness, irritability and anxious reactions in the presence of a child who is the same age as the aborted child would be.

Fourth, the duration of the above difficulty and pain will last for at least one month or more and may be delayed up to a time period greater than six months and, in our experience, may re-occur in cycles.

Charting The Pain

The basic concepts described above are the features we see most often and which motivate us to formulate a plan that will help a woman re-integrate her life towards wholeness and health. As helpers, we attempt to give full energy and integrity to understand and absorb pain without judgment. We believe that understanding doesn't require agreement or disagreement. We chart the pain and the symptoms so as to know where or how to intervene at any particular time that is appropriate (see Table 1, page 14). This is done by using the letters of the word "AFTER" to first understand the pain and, second, by formulating a counseling plan that is personally meaningful and agreeable to the woman. As we have seen, each letter of the "AFTER" denotes an aspect of the individual's personality: Actions, Feelings, Thoughts, Energy and Relationships.

Table 1
Charting the Pain

Symptoms	Possible Treatment
A. *Actions* and observable behaviors (Examples: hostility, misrepresenting self, making decisions, dependency, seeing consequences)	Assertive training, role-playing, charting behaviors, modeling, homework assignments.
F. *Feelings* and observable emotions (Examples: anger, sadness, confusion, grief)	Eliciting feelings, self-disclosure, increasing range of emotions, grief therapy.
T. *Thoughts* (Examples: memory, reasoning, controlling thoughts, forgiveness)	Coping imagery, rational-emotive therapy, charting, written and verbal expression of thoughts.
E. *Energy* level and physical self (Examples: lack of sleep, nutrition, diet, anxiety)	Relaxation training, meditation, charting, abdominal breathing and biofeedback.
R. *Relationship* and quality of contact with others (Examples: intimacy, forgiveness, marital or family difficulties)	Reconciliation, communication training, relationship building.

Each aspect is singular and yet cannot be separated from the others. A description is as follows.

The letter "A" in AFTER conveys the *actions* of her life experience, now called forth to be reflected upon. Some have been relegated to memory and forgetfulness from the distant past. They include the full range of behavioral actions and how these contributed to the abortion decision, and now are a part of the personality mechanism used to deal with the pain, sometimes in healthy ways, sometimes in destructive ways. Ironically enough, sometimes the behavioral action patterns that led to the abortion decision are invoked again afterward to help cope with it. Thus, if the patterns were negative and destructive before the abortion, the healing will likewise be hindered by them after the abortion (for example, compulsive behavior blocking out others' input, and chemical and relationship dependency). We can see how crucial it is to relate to and treat the whole person with an understanding of who she was, how she made decisions, and how she acted before the abortion. The pattern—unless therapeutically or spiritually interrupted and corrected—will continue, and she will be no better equipped to experience healing now than she was then to avoid choosing what came to reveal itself, in the long run, as intense pain. The action pattern is psychologically interrupted and spiritually corrected and directed when, by the grace of God, she allows that which has broken her to help transform her. To affect the woman's actions, the counselor may seek, in terms of goals, to lessen hostility, impulsivity (a single spontaneous act), compulsivity (repeated spontaneous acts), and personal irresponsibility. The counselor may also address examples of phobias, self-abortion (obsession with self), self-destruction, sexual performance and stress reduction (dealing with everyday tensions and pressures).

The letter "F" in AFTER speaks to the *feelings* or emotions that are experienced. The counselor attempts to have the woman call to mind feelings about self and others. She is encouraged, perhaps for the first time, to explore and express what feelings she may have: anger, sadness, confusion, etc. A full range of emotions is possible. Angry outbursts and expressions of guilt are accepted without judgment or control. In recognizing abortion as a major death experience, grief therapy is an important tool. This takes into account the stages of denial ("the abortion was no big deal" or "many women have an abortion and they get over it"), anger ("I hate God for letting me do this"), bargaining ("God, if you forgive me, I'll go to church every Sunday, stop smoking and be a better wife and mother"), depression ("I don't see any reason to keep living, I'll never feel any different than I do now"), acceptance ("I know what I did was wrong and God knows how deeply sorry I am. He forgives me and I forgive myself and now I can go on with my life").

The woman has a need and a right to display appropriate anger towards herself, others, and God about her abortion. The woman has a need and a right to grieve over the loss of her child, now seen personally and intimately. The woman has a need and a right to work through the emotions and words that, up until this point, have been confused and jumbled. When separated, the emotions and the words become better understood.

The letter " T " in the word AFTER is seen as the *thought* component of the woman's personality. The re-experiencing and the avoidance of thoughts, communication habits, the ability to understand cause and effect relations, and the uncontrollable recollections of the abortion experience essentially lie in the thought sphere part of the personality. The counselor can aid in focusing on the understanding of personal responsibility, forgiveness of self and others, and methods of psychological defense (rational thoughts that may lead to deeper insights into herself). Accepting personal responsibility (the fact that the abortion was rooted in the woman's own decision and thoughts) by the woman herself is at the center of the counselor's perspective. The counselor must be careful he or she does not read too much into the woman's thoughts and project onto them. Thus, the counselor enters into the world of forgotten events, concentration difficulties and hopes for the future.

The "E" in the word AFTER is related to the *physical energy level* that the woman sees in herself. She may see herself as functioning with a surplus of energy. Perhaps in an effort to keep very busy and stimulated with high sugar content food or prescription drugs, she may not have to stop and reflectively face her feelings. Conversely, she may function each day feeling very drained, energy for her body sapped by the psychological mask that must be kept in place to hide the feelings and thoughts that cannot be faced. The energy level needs to be brought back into balance so that her physical health can be restored. This is an integral part of restoring her psychological and spiritual health. Special attention should be given, when called for, to a balanced diet, proper rest, reducing potential dangers of physical stress, and dealing with other pain such as headaches, backaches, intestinal difficulties and other medical problems which may be the result of repressed post-abortion anxieties. For some people, physical pain is the cause of mental anguish. For others, it is the result. The aborted woman is most often among the latter.

The letter "R" in AFTER stands for *relationships* and it is, in our work, the most critical of the five components. The basic issues of human relational suffering present a particular challenge to the victims of abortion pain, especially when the woman has long pretended to the world around her that she belongs with friends, family and God when in actuality, deep inside the world within, she feels she does not. She struggles to increase or decrease personal contact and commitment, to engage in honest or guarded communication, to accept greater or lesser intimacy, enhance or dissolve marital and/or parental relationships and ask for forgiveness or deny the need for it. The personality and spiritual growth and conviction that is needed to choose the former over the latter of each of the above calls for specific psychological and spiritual goals that the woman not only recognizes as necessary, but to which she is also willing to commit herself.

Psychologically, the counselor can be of great assistance to the woman when he or she helps her see how she can communicate and relate with honesty, intimacy, and positive regard for others and herself. As a woman sees herself develop the ability to better handle responsibilities, ask for forgiveness when she is wrong (especially from children and those with less relational power and authority than she) and express positive emotional concerns and feelings towards others in an affirmative way, she comes closer to being an honest, intimate and communicating human being.

Spiritually, the counselor can likewise be of great assistance when he or she leads the woman to see that the realization of spiritual goals can liberate the human personality from the compulsions that often enslave it. Basically, compulsions are simply normal, healthy needs or urges taken to an extreme. For example, the need to be right and special, to be wise and faithful, to give, succeed, do and be settled, are in themselves good and healthy and yet can become compulsions when they are sought at all costs, without regard to any other values; either of self, or of others. Any of these compulsions has the power to affect the thoughts, feelings and actions of a woman to the point of an abortion decision. At the same time, the healthy expression of any of these needs is seen as part of the normal process and balance of accepting and handling the stresses of life, thus more likely precluding a decision that later would be seen as destructive and regrettable.

As the woman learns to communicate, trust, be truthful and empathize, develop a positive image of the world, herself, God and others, and come to accept herself for who she is and reality for what it is (and the abortion for what it means), she will most likely see her compulsions reduced to healthy expressions of basic human needs. This will enable her to be re-integrated into the faith community that is a part of her and accept the experience of God's love that calls her to be whole.

Having considered each of the five AFTER areas of concern, the counselor or clergyperson can then chart a planning/treatment profile that will be filled in and open to revision throughout the six stages of the healing process (see Table 2, page 20).

Table 2
Planning/Treatment Profile

Name: _____ Date: _____

Symptoms	*Possible Treatment*

Actions

_____

Feelings

_____

Thoughts

_____

Energy

_____

Relationships

_____

4.

The Counseling and Healing Process: A Holistic Approach

Each woman who is referred to us for counseling comes with a story that is uniquely hers. We, as her listeners, must integrate her story into our own life story. Our effectiveness as counselors is reflective of our own effectiveness in life. As friend to friend in counseling, we strive to put the pieces of information together in an effort to help health and healing become a reality. Hopefully, we can succeed in some manner in being free to learn to be healed ourselves without fear of having our sense of self destroyed. The open searching for insight and discoveries with a woman as to the meaning of her abortion will, in part, mirror our own willingness to honestly, gently, and with integrity find meaning in our effort to live our own lives with freedom and responsibility. Through this process she may learn that we all struggle to deal with life's stress-filled decisions each day.

This chapter has to do with how the information (experience, memories, hurts, etc.) of a woman's life can be organized and understood in such a fashion as to restore her to a state of integration and wholeness. Once healed, she is then able to function in harmony with herself, the world around her and her God. Her *Actions, Feelings, Thoughts, Energy* and *Relationships* will interact together and form a foundational harmony as spokes of a wheel radiating from the same hub. At the center of all this is the knowledge of who she is and the ability to feel good about this "new-found" knowledge. In a sense, she then feels she has it all together.

Theories of Counseling and Healing

The format and methods applied are generally known to anyone who has ever counseled on a therapeutic and/or pastoral level. What we've tried to do, however, is organize various approaches in a way that can be personally meaningful to a woman so that she may view the various aspects of her life as a whole, not as an indeterminate number of isolated symptoms. Thus, our approach is holistic and has its underpinnings in a variety of theories and techniques.

Relative to theory, for example, the term AFTER comes out of the work of Arnold Lazarus (1973) and his multimodal therapy (*The Practice of Multimodal Therapy*, McGraw-Hill, NY, 1981), a therapeutic approach which examines the various factors of human experience: a person's behavior, affect, physiological sensations, imagery, cognition, interpersonal relationships, and biological functioning. It is an approach of measurement that looks at the surpluses and deficits in each of the above areas so that specific treatments can be used for specific difficulties. In theory, human personality consists of all these factors. We behave, have emotions, experience physical sensations, think of mental pictures, create thoughts, associate with others and manifest biological realities such as sleeping and eating. Theorists of this approach believe that therapeutic change results from considering each factor and applying the appropriate research technique to the specific problems.

A second theoretical system is the enneagram. This is a recently explored system of spiritual investigations studied by John Burchhill, O.P., and Barbara Metz, S.N.D. de N., *The Enneagram and Prayer* (Dimension Book, Inc., Denville, NJ 07834, 1987).

Their work was based upon an earlier publication, "The Enneagram," by Maria Beesing, Robert Nogosek and Patrick O'Leary who have been working with this self-discovery model since 1974. The authors of these books have given retreats and workshops based upon the enneagram system that view personality styles as types of normal human needs that can have both healthy and unhealthy expressions. The unhealthy expression of needs manifests particular behaviors and affective avoidances with traps that prevent greater personal freedom. The healthy expression of these enable a person to experience the freedom of accepting imperfections, giving to self, seeing hope and showing self-responsibility. The enneagram is a system of understanding that is non-clinical, although we have seen it lend itself to diagnosis, treatment and evaluation plans. This system allows a person to see the attitudinal distortions in life that are based upon overwhelming personality type needs. These needs limit self-understanding and the healing of life's hurts. Although these needs give a sense of security and meaning in life, they, at the same time, can limit a freedom of choice and truthful knowing of self.

Knowing self within the enneagram system is accomplished by identifying one's needs, avoiding behavior, reality sense, thinking traps and healthier expressions of personality type. Although the reader is encouraged to review the text, previously mentioned, the table below will

Table 3: Enneagram Personality Types

Personality Type Need to:	Avoidances in Life	Reality Sense Based on:	Traps Preventing Free Choice	Healthier Expressions of Needs
1. Be Right	Anger	Shoulds	Over-perfection	Be Accepting and Optimistic
2. Give	Own Needs	Approval from Others/Respect	Over-seeking	Be Assertive and Self-affirming
3. Succeed	Failure	Appearance to Others	Over-efficiency	Be Cooperative and Truthful
4. Be Special	Ordinariness	Scripts to Play	Over-reasoning	Be Principled and Ordinary
5. Be Knowing	Emptiness	Correctness	Over-observation	Be a Participator and Share with Others
6. Be Faithful	Deviance from Norm	Apprehensions	Over-security	Be Self-trusting and Objective
7. Be Okay	Life's Normal Pain	Planning	Over-idealism	Be Speculative and Accountable
8. Be a Doer	Weakness	Control of Environment	Over-seeking Justice	Be Giving and Compassionate
9. Be Settled	Conflict	Harmony	Over-seeking Peace	Be Practical and Self-assured

present a partial picture of the enneagram system (see Table 3). This is a system, in our experience, that allows the individual to act by accepting the freedom of self, responsibility, choice and spontaneity.

A third theoretical system is the Myers-Briggs Personality Inventory. This system looks at personality in terms of the rate at which individuals express themselves, the manner in which they receive information, the manner in which this information is processed and how this information is displayed. In our work, we use the writings of Charles Keating, *Who We Are Is How We Pray* (Dr. Charles J. Keating, Twenty-third Publications, Mystic, CT 06355, 1987) and Chester P. Michael and Marie C. Norrisey, *Prayer and Temperament* (The Open Door, Inc., Charlottesville, VA 22902, 1984). The Myers-Briggs Personality Inventory itself is a test composed of eight different observations of personality preferences which are grouped into four scales. The first scale, Introversion-Extroversion, measures the manner and rate at which an individual manifests his or her personality. The second scale, Intuitive-Sensing, explores the style of receiving information. The third scale, Thinking-Feeling, involves the way in which information is processed. The final scale, Perception-Judging, determines how information, received and processed, will most likely be used. The eight observations of personality preferences can be grouped in various ways, sixteen totally different personality preference types may be seen in the general population. These characteristics of human personality, which in large part are built upon the work of psychologist Carl Jung, help individuals to understand and act upon their personality preferences in everyday life, thus seeing the healthy and unhealthy expressions of their attitudes and behavioral styles (see Table 4: Myers-Briggs Personality Types, p. 26). In addition, if they so choose, in post-abortion counseling, the preferences may aid

Table 4: Myers-Briggs Personality Types

Scales Of Attitude and Behavioral Style	Expression Tendencies	Unhealthy Expressions	Healthy Expressions
1. Extroversion	Acting/seeing variety	Over-control, aggression, may avoid weakness	Can enter into relationships
2. Introversion	Reflecting/ concentrating	Withdrawal, passivity, avoidance of relationships	Demonstrating indepen-dence, concentration
3. Sensing	Present and seeing facts, details,	Avoid seeing possibilities and change	Practical, matter of fact, concrete
4. Intuition	Future and seeing possibilities and expecta-tions new problems	Avoid facts and present realities enthusiastic, can see the future	Sees implications, insight,
5. Thinking	Principles, theory and analyzing	Avoid comparisons and feelings	Logical, ingenious, matter of fact can organize, take a stand
6. Feeling	Values, Relationships and appreciating	Avoids objectivity and over-loyal	Shows compassion, concen-tration, can sell and teach
7. Judgment	Being settled, deciding, planned	Tries to be perfect and is rigid in thinking, may avoid anger	Shows decisiveness, concentrates on essentials, plan and follow-up
8. Perception	Being open to change and unplanned	Avoids conflict and decision making, can be careless	Shows acceptance, curiosity and adaptable to change

women in choosing the spiritual direction they desire after working through their trauma.

Our diagnostic system is a medical model born out of the *DSM-III-R*. *The Diagnostic and Statistical Manual* of the American Psychiatric Association, commonly called the *DSM-III-R*, is a system of behavioral assessment that clarifies various symptoms of emotional mental difficulties into identifying conditions. This particular identifying conditions are matched with researched techniques.

Our testing includes primarily the MMPI and Rorschach technique, and occasionally, the Sixteen-Personality Factor Questionnaire (Cattell, Eber and Tatsouka, 1970), which give a comprehensive description of personality in terms of behavioral and emotional traits.

The MMPI (Hathaway and McKinley, 1970) is a heavily researched assessment instrument that has been used to predict psychological difficulties and treatment outcome. It is an accurate, reliable and valid tool to a counselor in practical problem solving and decision-making.

When, in our experience, the demonstrated stress appears to be quite significant, we administer the Rorschach technique (Rorshach, H., Hans Huber, publisher, Bern, Switzerland, 1948). The Rorschach technique is a test that uses ink blots, which can help the counselor determine the woman's style of coping; the difficulties in thinking that she may encounter, the rate at which she will function objectively, and be able to test reality and method of organizing perception and responding to the emotional aspects of her world. Psychologists and psychiatrists have used this test to tap the complexity of human psychological functioning.

Our techniques are primarily of a behavioral and structural family therapy nature, while being client-centered and encouraging the woman to act in acceptance of her freedom and self-responsibility. The behavioral goals and techniques translate therapy into action in life while at the same time allowing for freedom of choice, love and spontaneity. The family therapy goals and techniques explore the dynamics of relationship and communication processes.

As noted in Chapter 3, we chart the pain and symptoms a woman experiences by using the letters of the word AFTER to understand the pain and to formulate a counseling plan that is personally meaningful. Each letter of the acronym, AFTER, denotes an aspect of the individual's personality. Each aspect is singular and yet cannot be separated from the others with regard to the total person. A description of the counseling goals and techniques with respect to each personality aspect follows.

Goals and Techniques of the Counseling/ Healing Process

The letter "A" in AFTER conveys the *actions* of a person's life experience, now called forth to be reflected upon. Particular action goals have included:

1. Reduce aggressive behavior

2. Do not misrepresent self to others

3. Make simple and major life decisions

4. Perform life tasks attentively and with care

5. Increase exposure to anxiety situations and people

6. Change compulsive behavior (for example, alcohol use)

7. Reduce dependent behavior

8. Show willingness to seek reconciliation

9. Show satisfaction with self and others

10. Express interest and energy in work and non-work activities

11. Attend to life responsibilities

12. Display rational thoughts (for example, distinguish reality from fantasy, see consequences of one's actions, acquire insights and examine needs, etc.)

13. Show no denial of thought or feeling associated with the abortion

14. Complete exercises in letter writing, role playing, modeling, etc.

15. Participate in Baptismal ritual, prayer and Communion liturgy

Particular techniques that we have used in the action area include:

1. Charting personal behavior

2. Role playing and training of social skills

3. Assertiveness training relative to situations and need to change verbal and non-verbal reactions to individuals

4. In vivo assignments (for example, used to desensitize an individual's interactions that have previously been avoided)

5. Behavior reversal

6. Rational disputation of self-limiting thoughts

7. Coping imagery

8. Modeling positive behaviors

9. Anxiety management, including relaxation training, in the face of anxiety arousal

10.   Structured activities in post-abortion counseling and support groups

As noted earlier, the letter "F" addresses the *feelings* or emotions that are experienced. Particular goals have included:

1.   State feelings about self and others

2.   Display appropriate anger

3.   Display appropriate sadness

4.   Express separation between emotion and words

5.   Increase range of emotions

6.   Accept personal imperfections and mistakes

7.   Display fewer anger outbursts and reactions

8.   Report enjoyment of activities with others

9.   Cope with guilt laden thoughts producing guilt feelings

10.   Lessen startled response

11.   Complete grief therapy which includes experiencing denial, anger, bargaining, depression and acceptance— mourn the loss of the child

Techniques in the feeling area have included:

1.   Recording and self-monitoring of emotional expressions

2.   Elicitation of feelings

3.   Anger expression

4.   Self-disclosure of feelings

5. Anxiety management training

6. Relationship building

7. Rational emotive therapy relative to labeling, over-generalizing and catastrophizing

8. Repairing guilt by making amends

9. Overcoming shame through insight (acquiring a new way of seeing oneself) and conversion (identifying change in oneself)

10. Writing specific feelings relative to anger toward God for not intervening, toward themselves for their decision, toward others for their pressure and lack of support and information

11. Expression of grief and guilt

12. Written and verbal expression of forgiveness of self and others

Also mentioned in Chapter 3, the letter "T" in the word AFTER is seen as the *thought* component of the woman's personality. Particular goals have included:

1. Controlling thoughts relative to the re-experiencing and avoiding symptoms

2. Understanding cause and effect relationships

3. Reducing and eliminating intrusive recollections (non-controllable in origin, intensity or duration) and dreams of the trauma

4. Relating all thoughts relative to the trauma

5. Seeing hope for the future

6. Assuming personal responsibility, recognizing strengths and accomplishments

7. Recalling forgotten events and eliminating disassociative experiences

8. Maintaining concentration

9. Relating self-forgiveness and acceptance relative to personal meaning in life

10. Eliminating suicidal ideation

11. Demonstrating the ability to see the consequences of actions

12. Lessening the frequency of denial

13. Perceiving the child as real

Particular techniques we have used include:

1. Biblio-therapy and reading books such as the following:

A. *Daily We Touch Him—Practical Religious Experiences* by M. Basil Pennington, O.C.S.O. (Image Books, Garden City, NY, 1979).

B. *Reaching Out—The Three Movements of the Spiritual Life*, by Henri J. Nouwen (Image Books, Garden City, NY, 1986).

C. *Prayer and Temperament* by Chester P. Michael and Marie Norrisey (The Open Door, Inc., Charlottesville, VA, 1984).

D. *Who We Are Is How We Pray* by Charles J. Keating (Twenty-Third Publications, Mystic, CT, 1987).

E. *The Enneagram and Prayer* by Barbara Metz, S.N.D. de N. and John Burchill, O.P. (Dimension Books, Inc., Denville, NJ, 1987).

2. Rational discussion and acceptance of reality

3. Rational disputation (reasonable consideration of alternatives) and corrective self-thought of irrational self-talk (recognizing distortion in one's thinking patterns).

4. Organizing time, awareness training and seeing ahead of the present situation

5. Coping imagery (seeing oneself adequately deal with the abortion in a discussion with a loved one, friend or even antagonist)

6. Self-sufficiency assignments (goals to act upon with better functioning and adjustment)

7. Calming self-talk

As noted earlier, the "E" in the word AFTER is related to the physical *energy* level that woman sees in herself. Specific goals that the woman has formulated with us include:

1. Reduce physical effects of fear, anxiety and depression

2. Reduce insomnia or oversleeping

3. Stabilize medical difficulties

4. Experience fewer or no headaches

5. Engage in desired activities

6. Change semantic or bodily preoccupations

7. Change physiologic reactivity upon exposure to the events that symbolize or resemble an aspect of the abortion

8. Cultivate proper nutrition and rest

9. Develop meditation skills

10. Eliminate need for medication

Particular techniques in the energy component of personality include:

1. Recording and self-monitoring of bodily reactions

2. Relaxation training

3. Biofeedback

4. Abdominal breathing

5. Physical examination by the family doctor

6. Meditation exercise

7. Medication if warranted

Finally, the letter "R" stands for *relationships* refers to how the woman interacts with others. Relational goals include:

1. Displaying honest communication

2. Developing greater intimacy

3. Increasing exposure to anxiety-provoking situations with others

4. Handling personal responsibilities

5. Increasing personal contact with others

6. Following and participating in conversations

7. Expressing positive emotions and concerns towards others

8. Disclosing personal needs to chosen others

9. Recognizing the positive motivations of others

10. Changing parental relationships (for example, have the flexibility to request, persist, monitor, ignore, reward, encourage, compromise and penalize children when appropriate)

11. Changing marital relationships

12. Asking for forgiveness from oneself, the child and God

13. Participating in prayer and learning the process of reading, meditation, prayer and contemplation relative to the individual's personality style as indicated in the Myers-Briggs *Personality Inventory,* and explained in Prayer and Temperament.

14. Recognizing one's personal needs as indicated by others, relative to the enneagram

15. Experiencing the Sacrament of Reconciliation

Particular techniques that we have used include:

1. Role playing

2. Assertiveness training

3. Positive imagery

4. Family or marital therapy

5. Behavior rehearsal

6. Relationship building

7. Biblio-therapy

8. Discussion awareness exercise relative to spirituality

9. Reconciliation

10. Participation in post-abortion support group

11. Role-playing and letter writing with the aborted child

12. Giving the aborted child an identity and characteristics

13. Acknowledging the spiritual existence of the child

14. Acknowledging God's love

15. Encouragement of self-disclosure, inward probing and discovering of feelings, fluent and direct discussions, spontaneous sharing of self-experiences and display of greater self-respect

16. Discussion of self-temperament and needs

Stages of the Counseling/Healing Process

The sources of our referrals for post-abortion counseling generally come from the Project Rachel Community (a Catholic Church healing-outreach program), individual self-referral, physicians, clergypersons, and others in the mental health community. In a sense, counseling is both a science and an art in that the application of techniques depends on the counselor's insight into the possible correlation between specific problems and the needs of the woman that will best serve her journey toward health and wholeness.

A series of understandings of certain issues in the woman's life follows the initial referral. These are usually,

Table 4
Stages of the Counseling/Healing Process

1. Develop person to person relationship of unconditional regard and trust.

2. Reflect on past history of personal Action, Feeling, Thought, Energy and Relational status with possible testing and diagnostic assessment

3. Focus upon present Action, Feeling, Thought, Energy and Relational symptoms.

4. Review actual abortion events and processing of traumatic symptoms with regard to Action, Feeling, Thoughts, Energy and Relationship.

5. Focus upon present stresses as they relate to future concerns.

6. Reconciliation and spiritual vision.

but not exclusively, conceived as six stages of counseling and healing. During the first stage of the counseling relationship, the counselor immediately begins to absorb the pain with a compassion and conviction that the woman has been harmed. With the knowledge that the relationship deepens only with as much unconditional regard and trust as is present, the counselor invites the woman to implicitly share how she has been hurt and is still hurting at a pace that is appropriate to the trust level. There is neither condemnation nor condonement. The woman is given permission to share her story at a level that she is comfortable with, yet constantly invited to look deeper into the meaning, implication and consequences of her own story. Just as when driving a car an individual cannot go from first to fourth gear without damage to an engine so also a woman cannot go from no trust to total trust without damage to the relationship with the counselor. The wise counselor is one who solidly communicates that the woman being counseled is accepted as she is, yet invited to become more, step-by-step, rather than in quantum leaps. Thus, it is unrealistic to expect a woman who is totally negative to be transformed into an extremely positive person within a session or two. A realistic goal for change and growth will induce a more positive response and cooperation from the woman. Questions during the first stage may include:

1. What personal actions are you experiencing at present or, in other words, what are you doing too much or too little of?

2. What feelings do you experience throughout the day?

3. What thoughts are okay or not okay for you?

4. Describe your physical energy and health.

5. Describe your present relationship with others.

During the second stage of counseling, usually at the end of the first session, the woman is asked to perform one or more of three tasks, if she so agrees:

1. Reflect, during the next week, on her family, personal and relational history (this helps the counselor get to know her, as well as to see patterns of actions, feelings, thoughts and relationships).

2. Complete a DSM-III-R questionnaire immediately after the session or before the next session, if possible.

3. Schedule a time for some personality testing that will be used to provide further insights into her present difficulty.

The reflection on the woman's past history and present status may include questions such as:

1. What kind of person is or was (name a significant family member)? (This person is usually the first individual mentioned in the counseling process.)

2. How did others react to your abortion in terms of their actions, feelings, thoughts, etc.?

3. What has been or is their or your position on abortion?

4. How were you or they affected or "helped" at the time of your abortion?

5. How was the situation interpreted by significant persons?

6. What did or do others (that you know and care about) act, think or feel with respect to abortion?

7. To what extent have you experienced guilt since the abortion?

8. What has been the source of this guilt (family friends, religion, etc.)?

9. Is there any specific person in your life right now through whose presence, influence or opinion you would not have chosen an abortion? What is his or her opinion of you?

The DSM-III-R, a standard psychiatric-psychological interview assessment device, may prove helpful. Questions that essentially review the possible presence of any depression, variations in thought processes, anxiety and avoidance behaviors, delusions or hallucinations, or physiological difficulties should be asked. Women who have had an abortion may express anxiety and avoidance behavior (that is, resistance to any situation, circumstance or person that may trigger a recollection of the abortion). Some of the questions one may specifically ask include:

1. Did you or are you now experiencing any physical problems?

2. Did you or are you now experiencing any hallucinations or delusions?

3. Were you or are you now anxious about separation from those to whom you are attached?

4. Did you or are you now withdrawing from others?

5. Were you or are you now usually anxious throughout the day?

6. If so, do you feel the anxiety is related to the stress of the abortion?

7. Did you or do you now repeatedly re-experience the abortion?

An affirmative answer to these questions points to a post-traumatic stress disorder and post-abortion syndrome. Many women may wish to undergo further testing so as to obtain greater insight into their difficulty. Testing instruments include MMPI, Myers-Briggs, 16-PF and occasionally Rorschach.

During the third stage of the counseling relationship, one can focus on controlling the present distressing symptoms by using the AFTER model of intervention (see Planning/Treatment Profile, Table 2, page 20).

During the fourth stage of counseling, the actual abortion and the events around the abortion trauma are processed with regard to Actions, Feelings, Thoughts, Energy and Relational concerns. Possible questions include:

1. What were your actions or behaviors at the time of the abortion?

2. What were your feelings at the time of the abortion?

3. What were your thoughts at the time of the abortion?

4. What was your state of health or energy level at the time of the abortion?

5. What were your relationships like at the time of the abortion?

6. When did you actually decide to abort?

7. Who pressured you about the abortion?

8. Who would experience regret or distress (in a selfish sense) if you had had the child?

9. Who was the first to recognize your thoughts and feelings?

10. Who took sides?

11. What were the sides?

12. What did you do when sides were taken?

13. What would happen if you presently had control of your feelings?

14. What are some messages that help you give up control?

15. What feelings are or are not expressed?

16. When have you felt angry?

17. When have you felt sad?

18. When have you felt depressed?

19. When have you felt confused?

20. Who has noticed your feelings?

21. Who has noticed your feelings, but has not responded?

22. Who has noticed your feelings, but has made you feel embarrassed about them?

23. Who has made you feel better?

24. What do you do when expressing a particularly strong or meaningful feeling?

25. When have you told a person that you experienced such a feeling?

26. How did you and the father get along at the time of pregnancy?

27. What do you know now that you didn't know then?

28. How did you discover that you were pregnant?

29. Who had the greatest influence on you at the time of your pregnancy?

30. How were you hurried into making the decision to have an abortion?

31. What kind of support would you have liked to have had?

32. Where was the place you had the abortion? What did you think about it? How did you feel about being there?

33. What thoughts and feelings did you try to suppress or cover up?

34. Describe any anger, ambivalence, depression, or guilt you felt.

35. What forgiveness have you experienced?

36. Do you believe your child has a spiritual existence? If so, describe it.

37. Do you believe that you have a spiritual existence? If so, describe it.

During the fifth stage of counseling, the woman is helped to deal with present stresses as they relate to future concerns. Possible questions include:

1. Can you or he/they handle the issues in your life?

2. In what way?

3. What kind of actions, feelings, thoughts, health-energy or relationships are needed?

4. What do you usually need in these particular kinds of situations?

5. What do you usually avoid in these particular situations?

6. What level of fulfillment will sustain your relationship?

7. What level of comfort will allow you to participate in a situation?

8. What is your basic temperament?

9. What does healing look like for you?

10. If the difficulty continues, what will you experience in five years?

11. What do you want most in life?

12. Do you have someone who will listen?

13. Do you have someone who will affirm?

14. Who is there for you?

15. How would you like to follow through with your responsibilities?

16. What do people know about you?

17. What do people not know about you?

18. What do you want other people to know?

19. What do you hope they never find out about you?

20. How do you want to meet your needs now?

21. How would you like to handle problems "X," "Y" and "Z"—the major decisions of your life (e.g. marriage, employment, children, friends, etc.) presently or in the future?

22. What part does your belief in God play in your life?

23. Do you believe in a spiritual existence for yourself in the future?

24. Do you believe you will see your child within a spiritual existence?

25. What would you like to tell your child?

26. What feelings would you like to share with your child?

27. What do you think your child would want you to know and to feel?

28. How can you accept God's forgiveness?

29. What will you do after you have realized that you have been forgiven?

30. What challenges must you face in life as you experience *forgiveness?*

31. How committed are you to changing those things in your life that presently block that experience of forgiveness?

32. What must you do to focus your energy on separating yourself from past habits?

33. How must you face your inner fears, confusion and self-doubts?

34. Are you willing to pay the price for change; the price of limiting past negative modes of behavior?

35. How do you see yourself confronting reality now?

36. How do you see yourself overcoming the previous self?

37. How do you see yourself vindicated and changed, etc.?

In stage six, we will consider some of the criteria that are useful in best understanding when to integrate the Sacrament of Reconciliation or scriptural prayer experiences into the woman's journey of healing. This faith integration must be done in such a way as to respect the therapeutic integrity of the psychological healing process and the spiritual integrity of the faith healing process to the benefit of both. Both aspects complement one another, yet they are distinct.

Questions that we begin to ask include:

1. Is your "God image" positive or negative?

2. How do you feel about God?

3. How do you think God feels about you?

4. Do you believe God wants to forgive you?

5. Do you believe God can forgive you?

6. Can you envision a time when you will forgive yourself because God encourages and wants you to forgive yourself?

7. What specific spiritual gift would you pray for through God's healing of your life?

8. How would you like that gift to serve others after the counseling process has been brought to a reasonable closure?

9. What image of Christ is the most attractive to you: Good Shepherd? Light of the World? Babe of Bethlehem? Child teaching in the Temple? Jesus transfigured on the Mountain of Tabor? Jesus walking on the Sea of Galilee? Jesus confronting the scribes and the Pharisees? Jesus holding the little children on his lap? Jesus raising Lazarus from the dead? Jesus comforting those who mourn? Jesus condemned in front of Pilate? Jesus carrying his cross? Jesus crucified upon the cross in loneliness and nakedness? Jesus laid in the tomb? Jesus risen from the dead? Jesus ascending to the Father?

10. Why did you choose the image of Christ that is most attractive to you?

11. How do you see that particular Christ ministering or healing you?

12. Do you relate more to God as Father, as Son or as Holy Spirit?

13. Why?

14. Are you interested in exploring further your personality type with specific methods of prayer or particular styles of spirituality?

15. How does the enneagram relate to your spiritual life at present and in the future?

16. Can you recall times from the Scriptures when Jesus or other biblical characters expressed to themselves or to others particularly healthy indications of needs, thus allowing their humanity to deepen their spirituality?

These questions are not meant to be used in a rigid and methodical point-by-point fashion. Rather, when considered as a whole, they will become threads of thought, interwoven to re-weave the fabric of the individual's life story.

5.

The Counseling Response

Each of the three women described in this book had no pre-existing pathological difficulty prior to her abortion. They gave no evidence of a need for DSM-III diagnosis or a need for counseling intervention. At the same time, they were subjected to the normal stresses of life that produce particular patterns of coping that apply to every day life. Like everyone else, they were on a journey of discovering who they and the world were and how consciously to deal with these realities. Their wants, beliefs and fears were characteristic experiences common to all of us. You and I and those we love, or don't love for that matter, undergo the same. Like ourselves, they occasionally lacked the courage, knowledge or experiential capacity to withstand environmental and self-distress. Depressant temptations of life would over-ride what they knew somehow would be consistent with who they really were and how they really wanted to think and act. In a sense they, like ourselves, would abort an inner will so as to conform to economic, social, and conceptual demands. The familiar coping methods would not be easily dislodged in the face of unfamiliar distress and suffering. During the first stage of the post-abortion counseling, much of the pre-existing non-pathological styles of living described here would, in ing non-pathological styles of living described here would, in all likelihood, not be revealed. Nevertheless, at one time during the healing process, usually the fifth stage, the selfhood achieved prior to the abortion would come forth in discussion.

In this process, the distress of the abortion and its aftermath would be understood and give meaning to the present suffering resulting from the abortion. Hopefully, an enhanced psychological maturity would evolve in a personal source of life rediscovered. There would be a return to health with new knowledge and enhanced coping skills. The following examples provide the aforementioned sixth stage outline of therapy for each woman and take into account her normal personality, coping styles and post-abortion syndrome difficulty.

Helen

During the first stage of counseling, Helen complained that "all drive and life had been taken from her." Her pre-abortion style of coping with life had little meaning in the face of the abortion aftermath distress. Her present experience of self was of being "a failure to herself" even though she did the "right thing" in the eyes of her parents and husband-to-be and, yes, herself as well. She wanted to recover the sense of self that made her once proud of how people looked at her, and yet, at the same time, she had the disillusioned sense of experiencing shallow external evaluation by others which she somehow connected with her decision to abort. A dependency on achievement no longer had meaning, and she was hurt that "others didn't see her pain" and that she herself could not somehow rise above the abortion event.

She didn't want to be judged unhappy or filled with guilt. Having had her abortion during the second trimester, she had perceived movement within her and had had thoughts of the fetus as a human being. Her parents may have been correct in pointing out that this was the reason she felt so badly, but that was not what Helen wanted to hear. Although initially she had been satisfied with the abortion decision and in fact, relieved, perhaps as a result of her fiance's support, she now found little, if any, satisfaction in any relationship and was withdrawing from others. She thought her purported self image and future coping abilities would never be as strong as they had been prior to the abortion. Throughout the day she experienced an enhanced anxiety and a disruption in the sexual relations she had with her fiance. She was angry that the abortion did not reduce the anxiety of being judged. She wondered if she had ever been given emotional support by others. Having a child before marriage was thought to be immoral, so why was it now difficult to make other decisions in her life?

By the end of the second session, many of Helen's current actions, feelings, thoughts, physical energy considerations and relational issues had surfaced. Her ideal self was experiencing an ordeal and she had lost, for the moment, the positive source of life within her. She had been shocked by the abortion even though she had initially felt relief and, what was worse, indifference. She felt angry and chaotic relative to others and herself.

Well into the second stage, by the third session, Helen continued to reflect upon her past and present relational history. She began to organize her perceptions as to how others and she herself reacted to her pregnancy with respect to actions, feelings and thoughts. She began to discuss her thoughts and feelings about death, and how she would or would not be supported in her opinions. For the time being, she could not forget herself enough to think about a dead child and would vacillate between wanting and not wanting to have children. Her views would be respected.

Helen agreed to complete a DSM-III Structured Interview Questionnaire, MMPI testing and Myers-Briggs Inventory. When combined with the initial sessions, the result of these evaluations would help create a review of symptoms of distress and a treatment plan that could be modified at any time throughout the counseling relationship. Depending upon the severity of symptoms displayed during counseling and through testing, Helen may have also been given the Rorschach for the purpose of further determining her style of perception, control of emotion, stress tolerance and impulse control.

The DSM-III written interview revealed that Helen believed the abortion experience was a traumatic event, outside the range of normal human experience. Her difficulty occurred after one month and was characterized by recurrent and intrusive recollections of the building, abortion table and medical staff. In addition, she was presently experiencing a decreased interest in activities she used to enjoy. She also had insomnia and difficulty concentrating. Associated features included impulse buying behavior, instability, sexual dysfunction and anger towards God.

Helen's MMPI scores were similar to individuals who are impulsive, anxious and depressed. Particular critical test question items would be incorporated in the review of symptom questioning during the third stage and review of the abortion event of the fourth stage. An initial Profile Planning Chart was designed (see Table 5, page 53). Her chart would be reviewed, revised and updated throughout the counseling process.

Myers-Briggs inventory results portrayed Helen as someone who actively focused on possibilities with personal warmth. Similar individuals sometimes had normal difficulties being mindful of practicalities and facts and occasionally could be lacking in patience. These normal human traits would be reviewed during the fifth stage when examining the present coping skills and future considerations.

Assessment in counseling is, of course, an ongoing process and so we would examine personal needs and avoidances relative to the enneagrams schematic for the purpose of setting and trying out new actions, feelings, thoughts and relational goals. Helen, for example, would see and act upon her fear of failing, lack of trust in herself and her giving to others to prove herself worthy. Throughout the entire process and, in particular in the final stages, she would be affirmed in her effort to show equality in relationship, truth without justification, and dependency on reality. These are all aspects of a healthier manner of achieving a successful mode of behavior—a mode that does not depend on others to do one's own work and thinking, that is, one that does not demand repression of feelings and thoughts, and avoidance of conflict.

Table 5
Helen's Initial Planning Profile Chart

	Symptoms	Possible Treatment
Actions	Impulse buying	Behavior rehearsal
	Avoidance of conflict	Assertion training
	Dependency on others	Role playing
		Self-sufficiency assignments
Feelings	Anxiety	Elicit feelings
	Anger and grief	Grief therapy
	Fear of failing	Rational disputation
Thoughts	Thoughts of immorality	Positive coping statements
	Thoughts of death	Coping imagery
	Intrusive thoughts about the abortion	Rational discussion/ Thought-stopping
Energy	Decreased activity	Physical exercises
		Reassurance
Relationships	Sexual difficulty	Sex education
	Chaotic relationships	Communication training
	Pleasing others at all cost	Assertion training
		Rational discussion

Theresa

Theresa stated that her "present life had no meaning." During the first stage of counseling, she complained that there wasn't anything that she could be given that would enable her to overcome her sense of loss. She expressed the pain and hopelessness of not being able to do anything that could make a difference in her life. She thought she had sacrificed opportunities that could no longer be regained. Her familiar methods of planning and controlling her life no longer worked, and conscious control over experiences had a hollow ring. There was no amount or type of information that would bring comfort. She could not forget that she had had an abortion and resented not only the lack of control over her thoughts, but also the thoughts of those who were associated with her decision. She had tried to deny her pain by rationalizing "all women go through this for a short period of time—it's not so difficult—no one is to blame—look at the circumstances—I can't really be harmed by all of this—I just won't let it bother me." She fantasized, "it will go away," and minimized, "it's not all that bad." She projected, "it's not really my fault. Look at the way I was raised." She had repressive thoughts such as, "I can't bear to think about this anymore. I really don't even want to talk about it."

She wanted a quick solution to her discomfort at the time she came in for counseling, even before looking at the defined difficulty. As a result, she experienced depression and confusion. She could not confront the pain during the first stage, for she needed time to sort out her beliefs, understand and express her feelings and observe her relationships with others. At that time and throughout counseling, she needed a support system presented by one who was compassionate and could suffer with her in her loss. She was experiencing the inner tension that comes before the storm of identifying problems; she was challenging herself to confront the symptoms with the style and skill of relating to others as she used to deal with them in normal aspects of life.

She noted that abortion seemed to lower her self-esteem. She wondered if her conservative religious experience was adding pressure to her abortion experience. For the first time in her life, she had thoughts of suicide. She even looked temptingly at the sleeping pills in the medicine cabinet. What few close friends she had were concerned but felt put off by her aggressive attitudes. In fact, she seemed to be bitter towards men and, in particular, the father of the child. She was uneasy with these thoughts and just "couldn't understand how a procedure that should prevent the possibility of mental illness and disruption in life could bring the reactions that had occurred. What was it that brought about her reactions anyway, the lack of support of parents and friends, of clinic personnel? Why hadn't she been told of the alternatives, procedures and possible outcomes?"

On into the second stage, she judged that her decision was not easy. Later she would realize that the decision could have been affected by the thoughts and opinions of others. It appeared that her relationships had greater importance in her decision than did where she lived and how much money she had. Once angry at the unborn child, she now became angry at herself and others that she wished had helped to stop her and thus prevent a long standing trauma.

While in the second stage, Theresa completed a DSM-III Structured Interview between counseling sessions. She regarded the abortion experience as something that would go beyond any marital conflict, death, chronic illness or any other type of business loss. She likened the abortion to seeing someone shot or losing a limb or being trapped in a fire. She said that she would suddenly feel as if the abortion were going to occur again, whenever she saw an automobile accident or heard an ambulance with its siren blaring. At the same time, her feelings seemed for the most part anesthetized and constricted. With others she felt emotionally numb. She seemed not only to avoid feelings, but would also avoid any situation that would recall the trauma, such as a newborn child, pregnant women and driving by hospitals. Conflicts at work, relative to differences of opinion, somehow resembled the conflict around the decision making process when she was deciding to have an abortion. Understanding her feelings or even relating them would bring on memories of the abortion experience. She could still be logical, but was depressed and restless when hearing the emotions of others. She wondered if her increase in alcohol consumption was related to her discomfort. At the beginning of Stage 3, a Planning Profile Chart, that recorded alcohol consumption, was designed (see Table 6, page 57).

Theresa's MMPI score showed elevations in anxiety, depression and suspiciousness. Specific test questions relative to alcohol stress, family conflict and unusual thinking were examined.

Theresa's Myers-Briggs testing results showed her to be similar to individuals who were prone towards impersonal analysis with a focus on logic and theories. Similar individuals sometimes had normal difficulties being mindful of feelings. Her style preferences would be reviewed during the fifth stage while examining coping skills and future considerations.

Also, primarily during the fifth stage, Theresa would become more aware of her personal needs and avoidances with the definitions of the enneagram structure. New actions, feelings, thinking and relational goals would be created. She would, for example, see and act upon her tendency to over-seek security and be an idealistic observer of life. She would learn to trust objective realities and actualize her feelings and thoughts. She needed to control her fear of not knowing by being unself-conscious, undemanding and accepting of others and herself. No longer over-sensitive to rejection, she could relate to those whose views might be different from her own. Her ability to adapt to the world would be tied into being less analytical and serious about herself, and more approachable and balanced in the presence of others.

Table 6
Theresa's Initial Planning Profile Chart

	Symptoms	Possible Treatment
Actions	Aggression Suicidal ideation Re-experiencing event	Assertive training Removal of all medication Acceptance of reality Rational discussion

Feelings	Depression
	Anger, Emotional
	  numbness
	Over-sensitive to
	  rejection
		Effort to elicit all feelings
		Self-disclosure, Grief therapy
		Assertion training
		De-sensitization

Thoughts	Lack of thought control Confusion Lower self-esteem	Coping imagery Relaxation Corrective self-talk Self-sufficiency talks
Energy	Inner tension Alcohol consumption	Relaxation training Contract control and/or elimination
Relationships	Suspiciousness Controlling and dominating	Reconciliation

Ingrid

Ingrid initially talked about "being out of control." She didn't know what to do to discover and/or recover the sense of self she had enjoyed up to the time of her abortion. The immaturity of always trying to be "above it all" and of showing intolerance towards others was weakened and now a new way of showing compassion towards others was something she spoke of during the second session.

Throughout the first stage as well as during those that would follow, her assumptions and beliefs of how the world worked would be shared friend-to-friend in whatever terms she wished to use. Her personal story could be quite self-centered as may be the story of many her age. However, even though it seemed that she was acting on a stage and looking for affirmation about who she was, we would attempt to build trust by giving feedback and reflective listening during the initial stages of counseling.

As with other women her age, we would be aware of how she may not have had practice anticipating outcomes, seeing cause and effect, testing ideas, associating behaviors with results and overcoming immediate and overwhelming concrete demands. Attempting to feel a sense of personal power, she would perhaps later see some illusionary thoughts, such as we all carry during our journey out of adolescence. By the end of the counseling, she would perhaps determine greater differences between truth, falsity and fantasy. Ego bonds would be broken and self-hood already achieved left behind.

Ingrid noted that initially she did not have the same kind of negative reaction that a friend of hers had had immediately following her abortion. She wondered if the difference in initial reaction was because her friend had experienced emotional difficulties prior to the pregnancy and abortion. But now, they both seemed to be suffering in the same way. Why was this so? Both she and her friend were now of the same mind and said things to each other like, "I don't even think I can be a mother after what I've done."

Ingrid noted that her boy friend was currently feeling guilty and confused, especially after viewing a TV program on men's rights in abortion where each participant defended everyone's rights except those of the child. She was angered by his assertion of rights in her decision and angry at the child for entering into the relationship she had with her boy friend. At first she thought maybe it would be different if they were married, but given her circumstances, the decision to abort seemed so much easier—at least on the surface.

The DSM-III Structured Interview revealed Ingrid to be feeling as if she had been in some kind of terrible, catastrophic accident. She experienced recurring dreams and would often awake in a state of terror after seeing or hearing a child trying to speak to her. She was finding herself becoming detached from others while often thinking that something was going to happen to her. She found herself repeating, "Why didn't I just die and the baby live?" She was restless and irritable, and prone to headaches which had not been present before her abortion. At one time, she had a reaction formation response of being bigger than all of this and that it really couldn't hurt her, but this response, this way of defending herself, could no longer hide the pain. She wanted to have time to sort out her beliefs and preferences and dreams. She needed compassion, caring, patience and acceptance as indicated on her Initial Planning Profile chart (see Table 7, page 60).

Ingrid's MMPI scores showed elevations in anxiety and depression.

Ingrid's Myers-Briggs preferences would be reviewed during the fifth stage while examining her coping skills and future plans. With respect to her normal needs, she needed to see how she had avoided showing any weakness in the past, and now could find herself being more giving, compassionate and personally responsible for her own needs.

Table 7
Ingrid's Initial Planning Profile Chart

	Symptoms	Possible Treatment
Actions	Intolerant	Assertiveness training
	Self-centered	Corrective self-talk
	Compassion and and caring	Role playing
Feelings	Lack of control	Self-disclosure, thought-stopping
	Grief	Grief therapy
	Depression	Positive self-statements
Thoughts	Irritable thoughts	Coping imagery
	Over-planning	Rational-emotive therapy
		Biblio-therapy
Energy	Sleeping difficulties	Exercise and proper diet
	Headaches	Relaxation training
Relationships	Patience	Communication training
	Acceptance	Reconciliation
		Behavioral rehearsal
		Guided Imagery

6.

The Spiritual Vision: Grace Works Through Nature

The groundwork has been laid. A significant trust level has been created between the counselor and the woman who has had an abortion. A context or texture has been established for wholeness to take root and build. Much therapeutic progress has taken place and the spiritual dimension has been significantly addressed in the fifth stage (focusing upon present stresses as they relate to future concerns). Now the text and content can be sought. The heart of the healing process can be envisioned—a wholeness of body, soul, and spirit that brings an inner peace and an outward vision of embracing life. The environment has been crucial. As the old adage goes, "One must belong to become." The counselor has gently yet firmly established a safe harbor for the woman to trust and share. He or she has provided a place where she has come to see herself as a *woman* who has had an abortion; a person—feminine, real, seeking to experience the wholeness she needs, wants and deserves—rather than an aborted woman. She has processed many of the significant events and patterns of her life, including the abortion, what led up to it and what has followed. Her restoration and healing will come through her recognition of who she is—a child of God, still loved by God—despite what she has done. Healing for her has become the journey of discovering the goodness of who she is beneath the evil of what she has done. She is now prepared to experience spiritually what she has learned therapeutically: "I don't have to be perfect to be loved," without rationalizing or justifying her behavior. Perhaps her pain has been intensified by defining herself by what she has done: "My identity is rooted in that abortion." Now the counseling has helped her to see that the abortion decision is most likely a reflection of many other stressful life decisions made in a similar way. She now knows that her personhood transcends and lies beneath the many identities she had projected.

Piagetian psychologists speak of concrete operational thinking and formal operational thinking. The former is not able to easily grasp consequences, results and long range implications of given behaviors and decisions. The latter is. Frequently, the abortion victim has a history of decision making that is done in a concrete operational way. Add to this the elements of anxiety, fear, and impulsivity and the results are predictable: long range pain, regret and even sometimes dysfunctionalism. A woman who saw herself as basically "good" before the abortion now can't understand how she could do such a thing. A woman who saw herself as "bad" before the abortion may wonder how she could have sunk so low, but overall may just look back upon the decision as a logical consequence of a negative self-fulfilling prophecy. "I don't deserve a child." "I can't handle a child." "What I've done corresponds to who I am."

Henry J. M. Nouwen, a well known priest and spiritual writer, believes that all sin is ultimately rooted in an unresolved hurt or past pain. Indeed, you might even say that all sin is basically a denial of Genesis 1:31, "God looked at everything he had made, and he found it very good . . . ." When we don't believe this basic validation of our identity through God's creative love, we try to compensate, often using things, power, control and even violence to prove to ourselves and others that we really are okay. An anxious pregnant woman is especially vulnerable. If she has placed the validation of her identity in the hands and opinions of her parents, boy friend or husband and they demand the abortion as a prerequisite for accepting and loving her, she may feel compelled to comply to gain the support she needs to survive. Many loved ones often feel at the time that abortion is the most compassionate response to an unplanned pregnancy. We must understand this influence on the mother as well as the father of an aborted child if we wish to consider them as victims rather than as terrorists. Much could be said about the parallel feelings of the male whose child has been aborted. In recognizing the reality of the abortion for what it's worth, his pain, too, is real. As his denial is broken through, he may wonder how he came to deny his most basic parental instincts of protector and provider as his counterpart denied hers as life-giver and nurturer. It is beyond the scope of this book, however, to deal with the specifics of the male's healing journey. Suffice it to say that ultimately his healing needs are as real and intense as the woman's, though often suppressed longer, and even sometimes denied throughout a lifetime. The relationship itself may not survive the pain, however. As one young woman said to the father of her aborted baby: "You must grieve this loss with me or I cannot have you in my life. Even then, it may not be enough." It wasn't. They broke up shortly thereafter, as is often the case. The grieving may initially be for one's self and be riddled with guilt, anger, rejection and self-punishment. Later, the woman will grieve for the loss, the pain, the death—the baby.

The illusion of a false definition of freedom may also be part of the problem. The need to "be free" and "be in control" (whatever that means) is an inculcated and culturally conditioned goal of our contemporary society, necessary for self-fulfillment and happiness in the eyes and minds of many. So has the woman been taught and thus does she act. When the result is violence, and abortion in particular, we may not all be guilty but as members of the same society and the same family of humankind, we are all responsible.

Stanley Hauerwas pinpoints well the relationship between freedom and violence in these words from *The Peaceable Kingdom:* ". . .The very claim of freedom as a possession, as our achievement, is but a manifestation of our sin. We are rooted in sin just to the extent we think we have the inherent power to claim our life—our character—as our particular achievement. . . . Our sin is the assumption that we are the creation of history through which we acquire and possess our character. . . . Sin (is the) fear that we will be 'nobody' if we lose control of our lives. . . We must use force to maintain the allusion that we are in control." The types of control and the needs we seek to fulfill are part of the identities we create that can compound the normal stresses of life.

One of the ironies of abortion is that it may be the choice of one who sees it as a way to be more free, an expression of control and command over one's destiny and life. Yet in the healing process that leads the woman to retrace the steps of her decision and the experience of her pain and loss, several insights are revealed. She sees that her failure to discover the sacredness of her child's life has diminished her own, not enhanced it, and that the destruction of that human life has not brought healing to her own. She may even be angry at God because he hasn't saved her from herself. In the end, the decision that was made to bring resolution, peace and finality to a "problem" has done just the opposite. She may momentarily seem more physically free because of the decision, but psychologically and spiritually she is more enslaved than ever, even sometimes functioning as a psychological time bomb during the denial period.

Learning the Story

The clergyperson who collaborates with the woman's counselor must take the time to be briefed about her therapeutic journey to date, a journey which was charted throughout the first five stages of the counseling-healing process (see Table 4, page 36). It is presupposed that she recognizes the need for both psychological and spiritual support and that the counselor has helped her see how well they can enhance and complement one another. The counselor can openly ask her about her perception concerning her growth and struggles, ups and downs, during the sessions and in between, with the awareness that this will be shared with the clergyperson that she may be better helped. With permission of the woman, the planning charts, with symptoms and treatments, can be shared with the clergyperson. It rests on the shoulders of the counselor to pave the way for the next trust relationship: that between the woman and the clergyperson. He or she should especially be aware of traumatic life experiences, past rejections, fears, broken relationships, etc.

Having been briefed on all of the above, it would be helpful for the clergyperson to take a few days to pray and reflect on what he or she now knows about this particular abortion victim and to seek the enlightenment of the Holy Spirit that will enable him or her to best respond as God would wish. Perhaps, even at this point, it can be seen that an abortion was a predictable result of all that preceded it in terms of life events, attitudes, feelings, self-image and personal struggles. Generally, the predictable results have no psychological pathology. At the same time, in specific cases we have seen, there have been overwhelming significant past stresses.

Several studies, for example, now show that many aborted women were victims of sexual abuse as children. They, who were the victims of violence, now become perpetrators. How? Why? Does not this knowledge of the woman's history or of similar insights demand even greater compassion and commitment to help heal? No matter what the past, no abortion decision is ever made in a vacuum. It is born of influences, pressures, fears, agendas, plans and many other factors. Most women seem to feel it was the only option, the only choice possible. Friends and family, who could and should have provided the support to prove otherwise, failed to do so. An insecure and fearful woman was then even more firmly convinced that: "I am incapable of bearing this child, much less deciding who should raise it." Her right to choose was really not much of a choice at all.

We live in a world of extremes. "Choose your corner—your position—then fight to defend it!" The woman who has had an abortion is responsible for her decision and her recognition of that fact is needed for healing. Yet a compassionate spiritual vision must be one of hope—". . .There is hope for your future,' says the Lord" (Jeremiah 31:17), and of hospitality—". . .Christians are thus trained to be the kind of people who are ready to receive and welcome children into the world. . ." (Stanley Hauerwas) ". . .The birth of a child represents nothing less than our commitment that God will not have this world 'bettered' through the destruction of life. . ." (*ibid*).

Our desire to help heal others must start with an awareness of ourselves. God is free to forgive us to the degree that we have forgiven others. We block his healing graces by our lack of forgiveness. When we come to know ourselves well, we realize that we all abort God's will in one way or another. We create many identities to avoid true self and God. Selfishness, arrogance self-righteousness, and judgmentalism are but a few of the ways we do this.

When especially a clergyperson or counselor is in touch with this part of him/herself, this can help to predispose one to openness and understanding and the gift of unconditional love and presence. This is humbling, for now I am called to help another person, not because I'm better, but because I'm similar, perhaps even weaker. Friend to friend, sinner to sinner. One is then led to see that between condemnation and condonement lies compassion and conviction. The woman's healing process will not be served or bettered by condemning her as a person or condoning the abortion. Both extremes will only leave her where she was found: victimized and broken. But compassion for her and conviction that the abortion has taken an innocent human life can lead to her healing.

For many, the abortion decision was made possible through rationalization ("if it's logical, it must be right"—an abortion can seem like the most logical and "right" decision during moments of stress and anguish) and depersonalization ("It's only the 'product' of pregnancy—it's not really a person"). The destruction of a pre-born human life has come through the depersonalization of its reality. The healing of the mother's life must come through its reversal: the personalization of that pre-born human life. The personhood that was denied must now be admitted. Her brokenness has come through the violation of her maternal nature. God now seeks to heal her by working through her nature. Likewise, the world's brokenness came through the violation of human nature, created by God. Its healing in this age of the Spirit comes through an immersion of Christ's nature in our own. The sacredness that was denied must now be admitted.

The Child as Healer

We are firmly convinced that the main vehicle the Lord uses to help heal the aborted woman is the child she aborted. Before the abortion the mother is the baby's lifeline to physical life. After the abortion, the baby is the mother's lifeline to spiritual life. From a Christian perspective, throughout the healing process, the aborted woman, like the repentant Roman soldier, still stands at the foot of Calvary, mourns her child and sees the cross. Yet now she looks beyond that cross, sees the open tomb and knows that Christ has risen and her baby, too, will rise. As God, the Father, used the crucified Christ to heal an aborted world, so also does Jesus use the crucified child to heal an aborted woman. The recurring insight continues: "that which has broken her will transform her."

How did it all happen in the first place? The journey of faith teaches us in a compelling way that when we take our eyes off Christ, we lose sight of who we are to one another: Mother to child, brother to sister, friend to friend.

Our faith perspective likewise teaches us that we often face pain and regret in a unique way, for we do not simply try to erase and forget, overlook and deny. Secular writers and historians have realized this. As Professor William Brennan writes, "Only when we draw conclusions from the past is there hope for the future." We are a people of memory and feeling. That which has happened in the past, which is remembered in faith and celebrated now can radically affect who we are, who we become. We deliberately remember that Christ has died. The abortion victim needs to remember that her baby has died. In faith we proclaim that Christ is risen. She must believe that her baby will rise. With definitive hope we proclaim that Christ will come again, and when He does He will be carrying her baby in His arms.

As the grieving woman remembers, she begins to heal and personalize and teach us about the spiritual vision as it continues to take shape in her own life. Time and time again, the woman has helped us as priest and counselor to understand the power of the Gospel and the meaning of the Gospel that we have sought to proclaim. Throughout the past several years, these women have given flesh and form, feeling and personal intimate faith to the spiritual dream we've tried to hold out to them. For as the memory of their baby has become more real and the experience of Christ's love more present, they have taught us that healing and holding, reconciliation and reunion, remembering and dreaming, all go hand in hand to lead a grieving mother, not only back to the arms of her Father, but back to the arms of her child as well.

The fullness of our Christian faith tells the woman loud and clear that as a faith people of hope and hospitality, we find our roots in the Bread, the Book, and the Body—and God always invites us to come back to him and be a part of himself.

> The Bread is the Eucharist ("Then taking bread and giving thanks, he broke it and gave it to them saying, 'This is my body, to be given for you; Do this as a remembrance of me' " Luke 22:19). Jesus invites her to be nourished through the death he died for her and the resurrection he holds out to her. Whatever her hunger of spirit, the impoverishment of self that she now faces can be overcome by the Lord who wishes to nourish her with himself. In the Catholic tradition, she prepares herself for this through the Sacrament of Reconciliation, as stated in a previously mentioned book (*Abortion and Healing*, Michael T. Mannion, Sheed & Ward, 1986): "In particular, the

role of the priest in the Sacrament is to definitively proclaim God's healing to his sister in Christ. The priest is no better than she, for he, too, is a sinner. In fact, it is God's irony and choice that he uses the broken to announce his wholeness, the fellow sinner to announce the presence of him who was without sin. The healing power of the priest is not his own. Of himself, he has no power. His authority comes from the community of the Church. Thus he represents not only himself, but Jesus, the founder of the community whose healing word he bears. His authority to proclaim that healing is the carpenter of Nazareth, the Christ whose presence the community is to embody."

The Sacrament of Reconciliation provides a unique time in a person's faith history when Christ is encountered through the mediation of the church community and the priest as the ordained representative of that community. The priest, a fellow pilgrim on this journey of healing, is gifted with the privilege of welcoming the woman back into full union with the church community. He is much more a healer than a judge. He is a proclaimer of the Lord's mercy.

The *Book* is the Holy Scriptures, recounting the innumerable times that the struggles of God's people have paralleled her own. The cycle of creation-sin-redemption is God's gift to her here and now, his present to her in his Word. There is a little of Abraham, Isaac, Jacob, Isaiah and Jeremiah in most of us and a lot of Jesus in all of us, though sometimes hidden very deep within us. "All Scripture is inspired of God and is useful for teaching—for reproof, correction and training in holiness,..." (2 Timothy 3:16); "For just as from the heavens the rain and the snow come down, and do not return there until they have watered the earth, making it fertile and fruitful,

giving seed to him who sows and bread to him who
eats, so shall my word be that goes forth from my
mouth; it shall not return to me void, but shall do my
will, achieving the end for which I sent it" (Isaiah
55:10-11).

The Body is the Christian Community, the group of
followers imperfect and sinful, struggling and striv-
ing, who attempt to "proclaim the death of the Lord
until he comes" and call forth the presence of Christ
that may be buried deep in the hearts of some of his
people. These are the people of the various
denominations and traditions who seek to experience
Jesus through one another: "I assure you, as often as
you did it (cared) for one of the least of these brothers
of Mine, even the least of them, you did it to Me"
(Matthew 25:40); "Where two or more are gathered in
My name, there am I in the midst of them" (Matthew
18:20).

Many psychologists speak of repression and depression as
two of the most common mental illnesses of today. Repression: "Forget the past. It's too painful to remember. It's over
anyway. Done with." Depression: "Fear the future. Escape
from it. Grab on to the high of this moment. Don't let go."
Again, our faith leads us to a different response. For through
the Bread, the Book and the Body, we know that our healing
comes precisely in remembering, not to be further broken by
regret and guilt, but to be given hope by seeing the past
through the transforming eyes of faith. Even a profound
spiritual experience of being reconciled with the past would
be incomplete without the hope, assured by faith, that one
will be re-united with the child that was lost and is now
grieved and mourned. Reconciliation and reunion go hand in
hand. All this is possible through the resurrection of Jesus
Christ. That is the pivot event of our faith existence. "Christ
is now raised from the dead, the first fruits of those who have

fallen asleep. Death came through a man, hence the resurrection of the dead comes through a man also. Just as in Adam all die, so in Christ all will come to life again, . . ." (1 Corinthians 15:20-22).

7.

The Integration of the Psychological and the Spiritual

The counselor, psychologist or psychiatrist may have used many tools: the examination of past, present and future Actions, Feelings, Thoughts, Energy and Relationship symptoms, the Myers-Briggs Personality Tests, the MMPI (Minnesota Multi-Phasic Personality Inventory), or the Enneagram. If so, these instruments would have provided very helpful insight into the personality and history of a particular abortion victim.

Specifically, the Enneagram gives insight into nine unique aspects of human personality. If we are truly made in God's image, these aspects are nine faces of God's reflection and image of himself in his people; nine ways that he witnesses or images his presence in the world, ways that we can see and come to understand the sacred in one another.

Likewise, the Myers-Briggs Personality test reflects, in a sense, sixteen expressions of God's image of himself and his people. We do not see one as better than the other, but each as presenting a different side of our humanity. We are careful to make sure that our God is not too small. He can manifest himself through a variety and multiplicity of personality types. There is no one uniform Christian personality type. Yet there are numerous qualities well marked in Scripture (e.g., Romans 12; 1 Corinthians 12; Ephesians 4) that hopefully are found throughout all personality types. We find in one another what we lack in ourselves. As Father John Bartolucci says: "None of us has it all together, but together we have it all." We grow best through complementarity, not competition.

The Minnesota Multi-Phasic Personality Inventory is another useful tool, for it, too, gives us insight into the whole and functional kind of person the abortion victim perhaps once was, and still can be.

In using these various tools to better understand where the woman has come from, where she is, where she is going, we must be careful not to canonize one given personality type over another, for the woman's healing and wholeness will come precisely because she has embarked upon a psycho-spiritual journey to become who she is and who God created her to be. Hopefully, through therapy, she will have seen and remembered those times when her choices did not reflect who she was in a life-giving, other-centered way, but what she wanted in a life-denying, self-centered way. At the time she might well have thought that what she wanted was really what she needed, yet now she has learned that when we receive what we want, we sometimes create our own crosses.

A true sign that the spiritual vision is emerging from the psychological journey is that one begins to seek God's will instead of one's own. It is the moment when one recognizes that what God wants for me is really good for me.

The Christian community is most "whole" when those who have been most broken, now not only seek God's will for themselves, but also allow their lives to become conduits of God's grace for others; when their memories make them more compassionate towards those that have yet to make the journey that has been theirs. A deep sense of inner peace in the individual is the prerequisite for such a spiritual contribution to the community. It is born of a humility rooted in a deep faith conviction that our most precious gift, as Henry Nouwen says, is "one's pure being with us." In other words, my value is not rooted in what I do, but in who I am—to you, to others, to myself, to my God. This is an awesome insight for an abortion victim on her road to wholeness. In this process, the mountain of the ego has been leveled and the valley of the negative self-image has been filled in. With the smooth plain that remains, one is now freer than ever to see oneself as God sees one and to be a pure vehicle and vessel of his love and will to others. No motive other than deep, sincere love and concern for the other remains. There is no hidden agenda. The person is valued for who she is and who God has made her to be. It is "free love" in the best and fullest sense of the word. The woman has learned that she was not loved for what she did, but for who she is. Now that which she received as a gift, she can freely give as a gift.

How does the woman who has had an abortion get to this point? How can the clergyperson build upon the counselor's work and help it happen, with the grace of God? We believe it is best to begin this stage, Stage 6, where the woman is. How does she see herself now? How does she feel about the sessions she has had with the counselor? Breakthroughs? Setbacks? How is she different now compared to what she was when the sessions began in terms of Actions, Feelings, Thoughts, Energy and Relationships? How does her estimation of her present psychological status compare with the feedback the clergyperson received from the counselor prior to meeting her? How is her view of life, people, God and self changed since the therapy began? In a very real sense all that has happened therapeutically is a preparation for what now may take place spiritually. The therapy has helped the woman reach up and out—beyond her previous limitations, guilt, reactions, fears and inadequacies, yet she is still incomplete. Now she is ready to meet a God who wishes to reach down and around to embrace her, love her and use her very nature to help heal her. Then the Christ within her will be alive again—then she will be complete. This profound and personal experience of a healing God is not something that can be forced upon her. It is built on God's grace and her response to it—called forth from her. It comes at a time when her whole definition of God may have changed from harsh and judging to loving and merciful. It comes at a time when she is attracted to God because she is drawn by his love rather than repulsed by fear of his punishment. It comes when she feels about God the way she now knows He feels about her. She now is sure he wants to forgive her and she holds the key to that forgiveness. God has already done his part on that dark but good Friday. Her faith has reached the point where she now has given herself permission to forgive herself, based on the tradition that comes to her through the Bread, the Book, and the Body. Now, she can even look beyond the present crisis and envision spiritual gifts that will be born in her from this loss. Already she senses she is more compassionate and understanding since she has experienced the forgiveness of a loving God, a forgiveness that she did not merit or deserve, or achieve but only came when she was finally ready to humbly accept it as gift. Already she senses a hunger in herself to serve others—not to atone for the guilt of the past, but to celebrate and give thanks for the free gift of forgiveness in the present.

The over-riding recognition that the author of life is the one who must heal the loss of life permeates the healing process. The Helen of Chapters 3 and 5 is no exception to this rule. The therapy revealed that she saw herself as one driven to achieve, insecure in decisions, feeling the need for perfection, to be loved and forever basing her decisions on others' anticipated reactions, thus always needing the approval of others. Her spiritual growth might be aided by her identification with the portrait of the Jesus who loved people for who they were, though imperfect; reassured the frightened and insecure; and led his disciples to ultimately listen to only one voice—that of the Father—as they sorted out decisions and options that confronted their lives each day. This biblical portrait of Christ might come through numerous scriptural stories and accounts:

• Jesus as the babe of Bethlehem (Matthew 2)—totally dependent on those around him and the Mary who bore him.

• The Child in the Temple (Luke 2)—teaching about the Father even as his parents sought him.

• The Messiah baptized by John (Mark 1)—publicly accepting his destiny to do the Father's will—unto death.

• The Prophet in his home town (Luke 4)—determined to preach, yet rejected by his own.

• The healing of his own and strangers (John 5)—expressing the Father's love for *all* his children.

• The Transfigured Lord (Mark 9)—empowered the more to face Jerusalem.

• Facing the Pharisees (Luke 5)—confronting those teaching evil masquerading as good.

• Blessing little children (Mark 10)—revealing them as the heart of the Kingdom of God.

- Mourning his friend Lazarus (John 11)—expressing the humanity and depth of his grief.

- Condemned by Pilate (Mark 15)—free not to be baited to hate.

- Crucified (Mark 15)—dying for all, even for those who killed him.

- Risen from the dead (John 20)—proving that "God's Kingdom comes not in spite of evil, but through it.... Goodness suffering to absorb evil and by doing so to redeem it."[1]

- Ascending to the Father (Luke 24; Acts 1)— Embraced by the Abba whose will he obeyed.

In this spiritual identification, Helen might even be led to know God's love through a centering prayer experience (explained in an excellent book by Basil Pennington, O.C.S.O., entitled *Centering Prayer* [Image Books, Garden City, NY, 1982]). In this beautiful prayer form, one: 1) *reads* the given Scripture passage, slowly and peacefully, perhaps several times; 2) *meditates* on the passage, reflecting on the power, meaning and sense of what's happening, perhaps even placing oneself in the story, at that place and time; 3) *contemplates* the presence of Christ, allowing his love to be felt and savored without the mediation of any particular images, thoughts or words (listening and feeling—not speaking and thinking); and finally, 4) *prays* that this experience of Christ might become a part of one's self and one's life.

The Theresa of Chapters 3 and 5 is loyal and conventional, the first-born and responsible, yet often rigid even to the point of believing that flexibility equals instability. Feeling that she has no right to enjoy life unless she figures it out, Theresa may hide behind the mask of domination and control when her security is threatened by situations demanding more flexibility than she feels she is able to tolerate. It is not difficult to see how an unplanned pregnancy—and the flexibility that would be required to bring a baby to term—could easily result in a dominating, take-control, not too well thought through, decision to abort. This is a Theresa who could better understand the past and learn from the future as she reflects upon a God who will give her strength to handle the unexpected and who promises ". . .all things work together for good to those who love God. . ." (Romans 8:28). She may well like to admire and try to identify with a Jesus who was constantly thrown into new situations and saw them as opportunities to serve the Father rather than as underlying crises to avoid others' judgments.

The psycho-spiritual healing process after an abortion is not just one that should bring reasonable closure to the abortion trauma, but one that will impact upon future decisions and perspectives of reality. It should help one see not only the past differently, but the future as well. Life hence should be viewed as an experience to be lived rather than as a battle to be won. In the lives of those abortion victims with particularly painful and even violent histories, one might even look back and see that she who was insecure about her own right to life could hardly bestow that right on the unborn child. Reflection and perspective, both psychological and spiritual, are two lessons born of adversity.

The Ingrid of Chapters 3 and 5 is one whose parents desperately needed her acceptance. Her childhood was a constant example of her taking advantage of their vulnerability. Weakness is to be avoided. Domination over peers is common. This requires being in control, even at the expense of friendships and loyalties, gentleness and tenderness. Her intentions to help others plan their futures through attentive listening are always good, yet truncated by her inability to plan for her own. Her moral maxim: "If it feels good, do it" has not brought her happiness. The present might momentarily carry her on the crest of a high, but before long, she comes crashing down.

There is a Jesus who leads by love and respect, rather than by power and domination; by invitation rather than subjugation. If Ingrid could accept and follow him, she would undoubtedly not only be freed from the compulsion to validate her worth by being in control, but would also see healthy qualities of leadership and personality emerge, previously submerged beneath her insecurities. This is the Christ of Matthew 4, whose eyes pierce the souls of Simon called Peter, and his brother, Andrew, when He says, "Come after me, and I will make you fishers of men" (19) and who then calls the others as well. They soon learned that they were not called for themselves only, but to lead others to the Kingdom. This is the Jesus of John 21:15-18 who still loved the same Simon/Peter three years later, after Peter's triple denial and his own crucifixion; who loved him to the point of entrusting the mission of the Kingdom to him once again: "Simon, son of John, feed my lambs. . . tend my sheep. . . feed my sheep." So, too, through reflection and perspective on the spiritual journey, do the Ingrids learn that they are healed, not only for themselves but to help strengthen others, once they themselves are strong.

The Enneagram and/or Myers-Briggs Personality Inventory can be of great help to the clergyperson as he or she builds upon the therapeutic process and leads the aborted woman to chart her own spiritual waters for the future, learning from the past as well. The counselor can brief the clergyperson on the woman's particular personality type or attitude and behavioral style and then help her pinpoint the distortions the type is prone to, that she specifically has experienced. Through this process, she learns she is not bad, but that the channeling and direction of her given personality must be positive. The personality type, in itself, is neutral—its expression can be positive or negative. Finally, God's grace works through her nature when the clergyperson helps her draw scriptural parallels and examples from biblical role models whose lives emulate the qualities, virtues and healthy need expressions that correspond to the given personality type. The examples follow:

Table 8:
Enneagram Personality Types
and Biblical Role Models

Personality Type Need to:	Healthier Expression of Needs	Biblical Role Models
1. Be Right	Be accepting and optimistic	**John 3:** Nicodemus hungered to be right and then learned the love of Jesus for the world and him was the bigger picture.
2. Give	Be assertive and self-affirming	**Ruth 1,16:** Ruth would not abandon her beloved Mother-In-Law, Naomi, even when others thought it best. ". . .wherever you go, I will go. . ."
3. Succeed	Be cooperative and truthful	**Luke 18:17:** The rich young man learns that real success is being true to one's self through God's call.
4. Be Special	Be principled and ordinary	**Matthew 15:21:** The common Canaanite woman sees her daughter healed through an unyielding faith that goes beyond logic.

5. Be Knowing	Be a participator and share with others	**Luke 9:46:** True wisdom is found in the childlikeness of one who comes before the Lord as he-she is, no illusions, no pretensions.
6. Be Faithful	Be self-trusting and objective	**Mark 2:23:** Jesus teaches about priorities: "The Sabbath was made for man and not man for the Sabbath."
7. Be Okay	Be speculative and accountable	**John 12:20:** Jesus teaches that life has meaning only when we die to self like the grain of wheat, not seeking pain for its own sake, but accepting it for its power to transcend and redeem.
8. Do	Be giving and compassionate	**Luke 23:32:** True strength and freedom is found in the power to be gentle and loving, even in the face of opposition and violence.
9. Be Settled	Be practical and self-assured	**Matthew 12:38:** Reality has to be faced. Compromise may only mean greater conflict later.

Table 9
Myers-Briggs Personality Types and Biblical Role Models

Scale of Attitude	Healthy Expression and Behavioral Style	Biblical Role Model
Extroversion	Be relational with reflection and knowledge of consequences	Moses (Exodus 33)
Introversion	Be independent in one's action	Jeremiah (Jeremiah 1)

Sensing	Be practical with awareness of self and others	Peter (John 21)
Intuition	Be insightful and giving	Paul (Romans 12)
Thinking	Be logical and knowing with faithfulness and loyalty	Nicodemus (John 3)
Feeling	Be compassionate with reasoning and principle	Zacchaeus (Luke 19)
Judgment	Be decisive with a sense of openness	Canaanite Woman (Mark 7)
Perception	Be open and spontaneous with closure and accountability	Micah (Micah 6)

The woman now sees more clearly how her God-given and naturally expressed characteristics and traits, qualities and habits can be integrated into spiritual goals and values, not alien, but basic to her. We can all learn from this that the true measure of a person is found in whether or not one can live and be true to one's own words. The Enneagram and its spiritual parallels should, by no means, discourage a woman in her psycho-spiritual healing process, but encourage her to see that there are concrete and practical ways that the holistic healing of body, soul, and spirit can become a reality for her.

Note

1. *The Hidden Years*, a novel about Jesus by Neil Boyd, (Twenty-Third Publications, Mystic, CT, 1986).

8.

The Celebration of the Psychological and the Spiritual

She has been struggling to forgive herself, and to allow God to forgive her. In the midst of the healing journey, she has begun to "feel good about herself," and to realize that the real issue spiritually is not the abortion, but *faith.* This is true of virtually any alienation from God. As mentioned previously: "Do I believe God *can* forgive me? Do I believe God *wants* to forgive me? Do I believe God *will* forgive me?" The spiritual healing and psychological wholeness will happen only when she reaches out to take the gift that God offers her. She will become humble and contrite, now sensing from within herself, rather than through the words of another, that, "The Author of life is the one who must heal the loss of life." She must challenge herself: "Will I allow God to give me permission to forgive myself? Will I accept his authority to heal me? Will I believe in that authority?" Many of us grow up never doubting God's power and authority to condemn, but are apprehensive about his authority and even his willingness to forgive. Even the events of our daily lives mirror such an attitude. An earthquake or a bolt of destructive lightning is an "act of God." The sunrise and the birth of a baby is "nature" and "human nature." We sometimes see God as we see ourselves—more inclined to believe the worst than the best.

"A boy friend has pushed me away, a parent has pushed me away, my friends have pushed me away, why will God be any different?" she wonders. Recently, a young father of eleven children, some adopted, some handicapped, some bi-racial spoke of the day he punished one of his children by confining him to his room for several hours. Lunch time came and the child insisted on sitting next to his father and holding his hand, totally secure and sure that his father would not let go and push him away. The father, with tears in his eyes, recounted what his child that day had taught him about God, his Father. He prayed that when he died his heavenly Father, though he had sinned many times and "been sent to his room" during life, would not withhold his hand and push him away at the heavenly table. This father of eleven always lets his children know that although they may "do bad things," they are not "bad." Our heavenly Father wishes to assure the woman who has had an abortion of the same truth: He won't pull away.

The woman of the Protestant tradition will find much comfort in praying with her minister or friend in faith. She can briefly recall her sessions with the counselor and what she has learned about how and why she came to choose an abortion. If she wishes, she can share the memory and the pain of it. She can explain how she felt about herself then and her doubts about God's love. She can share convictions about the reality of his love now. She no longer needs to rationalize—she knows her admission of responsibility is integral to her healing. She is ready to personalize: name her baby, describe her baby, pray to her baby for forgiveness.

The abortion was a statement of a mother's rejection of her baby. As a woman names her baby and says, "You are mine, I love you," she may in her heart of hearts hear her baby claim her as mother. The baby she has rejected now accepts and claims her as mother. There is a healing in this alone. These moments may well be among the most tender and tearful of her life. And the tears will be those of healing. Through the power of God's love, she believes in his forgiveness and her baby's forgiveness of her. She is empowered to forgive all those who, by voice or silence, action or absence, participated in the death of her child: father or mother, boy friend or husband, brother or sister, friend or physician. Sometime they, too, will have to come to grips with their role and their pain, even if now hidden and submerged, but her healing is not contingent on theirs.

God is free to heal who, when and where He wishes. She seeks to be as free to forgive as was Jesus from the gibbet of the Cross (Luke 23:34). Her freedom will bring the clear light to see her child in Jesus' arms, loved and wanted. Reconciliation has come now. Reunion will one day follow. This is God's promise (1 Thessalonians 5:13). Together, woman and friend may search the Scriptures and share those passages that have special meaning, times when God reached down to embrace His hurting people as they reached up and out in their pain. Through the psychological journey, the woman has reached up and out.

Through the spiritual journey, she has felt God reach down and around her. Grace has worked through nature. Grace embraced nature in a radical new way, when the angel Gabriel said to Mary: "Rejoice, O highly favored daughter!" (Luke 1:26). And she conceived of the Holy Spirit. Now that same grace of Christ comes to heal nature—her nature. The warmth and hospitality of many Protestant denominations has much to offer this woman, now needing and well-deserving of all the support a Christian community can give through worship, prayer and service.

The woman of the Catholic tradition can anticipate the celebration of the Sacrament of Reconciliation and the reception of Jesus in the Eucharist.

She can pray her life may echo by these faith celebrations the words of St. Paul: ". . .the life I live now is not my own; Christ is living in me. . ." (Galatians 2:20). Her need and hunger is for a personal relationship with Jesus. As Yahweh in the Hebrew Scriptures mediated his presence through the parting waters of the Red Sea (Exodus 14:10), the consuming fire on the mountaintop of Sinai (Exodus 24:12), and the gentle whispering sound around the cave of Horeb (1 Kings 19:9), so has he now in the New Covenant, sealed in the blood of his Son, mediated his presence through bread, wine, oil and water. It is Jesus saying: "Come to know me and be a part of me in the breaking of the Bread, and the Sharing of the Cup and the living of the Word" (John 6:52).

She is invited by the Church to prepare for this Bread of Life through the Sacrament of Reconciliation, through which she may be reconciled with the Lord in his Community, for the Church, too, is impoverished by the destruction of one of its own.

Days before the Sacrament is celebrated, the woman can choose a passage from the Scriptures that is particularly significant, perhaps one that has been previously shared in the Enneagram or one that expresses a Merciful Father (Psalm 130), a Healing Jesus (Luke 8:40), a Consoling Spirit (Galatians 4:1). There are many strong and very human Biblical faith figures among the women in the Scriptures: Sarah, Ruth, Esther, Deborah, Judith, Mary, Elizabeth, and Mary Magdalen, to name a few. She may wish to choose a passage that helps her identify with one of these women of faith. The timing of the Sacrament of Reconciliation and the reception of the Eucharist may be planned to coincide with dates that have special meaning: Christmas, Easter, the child's projected birth date, the mother's birthday—all appropriate times to celebrate new spiritual life, rebirth and renewal. Both these spiritual events are the church's way, in the spirit and footsteps of Jesus Himself, of saying: "Come back, Welcome home, You are wanted, You are loved."

The celebration of the Sacrament should include the Scriptures the woman has chosen and prayer to the Lord to receive her child into His arms. She may even want to read a letter to her baby, asking forgiveness, sharing her love. Her grieving process will find solace through her faith. As guilt subsides, the woman is more free to grieve and receive God's love for her as well. The greater the admission of sorrow and regret for our sin, the freer the Lord is to forgive us; the more open we are to accept his forgiveness. Through the Sacrament, she not only draws closer to her God, but to her child as well. Her willingness to grieve for her child has allowed the Lord to use her baby to lead her back to himself.

"Christ has died, Christ has risen, Christ will come again"—the Church has proclaimed since the early centuries. The Sacrament of Reconciliation reminds her that a daily identification with the death, resurrection and future reunion with Jesus will help her spiritual journey continue and grow. As her life conforms to the "dying to self" cross of Christ, her life will be transformed by the resurrection of Christ. The priest can further help her by asking how she wishes to live out that identification with the Paschal Mystery of Jesus in her life, and suggest a penance that corresponds to that wish. The sin was not trite, nor should the penance be. The woman would not be served by such a penance. The penance is not to intensify guilt, nor can it compensate for the past. It can and should be a way the woman tells her

God that she now wishes to be a life giver, following in the path of Jesus who came as Way, Truth and Life.

The Church, rooted in the teachings of Christ, has thought her pain and hurt serious enough to ritualize its resolution through the healing power of Christ in the Sacrament. This, too, should bring consolation.

A very special moment takes place when the woman shares in the Eucharist and receives the Body and Blood of Christ at Mass. The Lord she now receives is the Jesus who holds her child. An awareness of this can help her draw closer to her baby, lost physically, with her spiritually. The Lord of life, through his death and resurrection, transcends life and death, space and time. Those barriers no longer separate. God's people are not divided. We are one, through Him, with those who have gone before us "marked with the sign of faith." A woman may never feel closer to her child than when she receives the Eucharist.

Signs of Healing

The psychological and spiritual healing that should lead to an abortion victim's wholeness will reflect not just how she views the abortion of the past, but how she embraces the future. There are several signs that the healing is real for her, that she has integrated what she has learned: the unborn child, her vision of herself, her determination to remain true to innate instincts and decisions, her relationship with God, her understanding of intimacy and love.

The healing is real when she recognizes the mystery of God's gift of life and that a child's life is no less sacred because of the manner, timing or place of his or her conception. This healing is the God given integrated experience of using past memories of painful brokenness as a constructive lever to rebuild the future, rather than as a crutch to avoid it or remain dysfunctional or paralyzed by it.

This healing brings the freedom to be oneself and the maturity to live commitments with those who accept, enhance, and complement those commitments.

Healing is present when tears come not so much because the past is painfully remembered, but because the present now carries with it the Father's hope and love.

James Baldwin once said: "One cannot deny the humanity of another without diminishing one's own." These pages are testimony to the truthfulness of that statement, but more importantly, to the courage of the women who have grieved and mourned, dreamed and believed and, through it all, learned that the words of Jeremiah *do* apply to them:

Thus says the Lord:
In Rahmah is heard the sound of moaning,
of bitter weeping!
Rachel mourns her children,
she refuses to be consoled
because her children are no more.
Thus says the Lord:
Cease your cries of mourning,
wipe the tears from your eyes.
The sorrow you have shown shall have its reward,
says the Lord,
They shall return from the enemy's land.
There is hope for your future, says the Lord:
"Your sons shall return to their own borders"
Jeremiah 31: 15-17

There is hope for your future, says the Lord.

Appendix:
Personal Witnesses

The following personal witnesses are taken from the stories of three persons from three different countries. When read carefully, they reveal many of the principles discussed in this book.

Benjamin, Stephanie

Benjamin—Ben, I would call you
Stephanie—Stevie, I like that

Beautiful babies, the first Ben, you are pretty, like your father. Sensitive eyes blue, but later greenish brown and brown hair. You loved me and reached for me. I never meant to be a cold inhumane person. I thought my motherhood would always dominate but it was absent; you needed warmth, I gave you none. I was like a sick wicked girl condemning you in the process of your attempt to grow; I starved you. It was then I walked spiritless and God took you baby and kept you warm. He carried you, he held you and Mary held you as a mother should. You got love after the horrible pain. I'm so sorry please please forgive me for my weakness, my painful punishment that I gave you so undeservingly—too undeserved to speak of, my breath leaves me. You are my beautiful angel and saint. You were in a dream somehow just cognitively you made me aware that you are the strong peacemaker. You would have aided me in sorrow, please aid me now. Your strength baby it overwhelms me, love me, somehow pray to Jesus and ask him if when I die I can hold you and you will say "This is my mother." Ask Jesus to strengthen me in this stressful hard time. Benjamin, I didn't like that name, but somehow it came to my mind, Benny, Benjamin, Ben. Your middle name is Matthew. This is a beautiful name. You are a beautiful child. Always be happy, I will pray to you each day. All the love in my heart is for you baby. I will never forget you my first son.

This is so hard, God help me.

Stephanie Victoria, Stevie, like the uniqueness of your face I see. You have my dark hair, you face is tan and healthy and your eyes are blue. I feel them staying very blue. Baby girl I wanted to keep, when time allowed me to think. When you were inside me I felt so happy, like a mother. Remember my driving and talking to you? You are my precious girl. If I could only open my body and lift my heart up to give love to you and your brother, I would. I would love nothing more that to be your mommy right now; to walk you across the street holding hands. Baby please feel love in your heart for me. Make me feel it, tap my heart and cover me with warmth. You are a gift from God, created for me for a reason. I interfered with destiny, your's and your brother Benjamin Matthew's—I love you both. Help me to reach you both. Do you love each other's company? Is our God the most compassionate and warm of anything on this earth you see? (Yes) I know he loves us all; help me feel worthy of Him. Stephanie thank him for taking you into his arms. Your lives are so beautiful in heaven I'm sure. You have Grandfathers to love, who love you very much. They've kissed me, please kiss them so I can feel that I've kissed you both. Babies, I pray to join you. Please pray for me that I may see you someday and that I am fit to see our glorious father. Steph, I'll hold you someday too.

Birthdays: Benjamin, October 1986
               Stephanie, September 1987

April 3, 1988

Almost a Year Ago

I found out almost
a year ago
that I was pregnant with you
And, although I was scared. . .
so scared and so confused,
it was, at the same time, one of
the best feelings I had ever known. . .
to know that you were growing
inside of me—
because everything you represented
to me was good . . . hopeful
your innocence and your beauty
your potential as a person.
You represented the love that was (is)
shared between your father and me
I remember sitting in my room . . .
alone, in silence
I'd put my hand on my stomach
and I'd think about
　　what you would be like
　　　　what you would look like
Would you have a gift for writing
　　　　like your father?
　　Would you like baseball
　　　　and music
　　　　　　and puppies?
I'd think about days with you
in the sun,
　　　　me, you, and your daddy
laughing and playing together
in the sand near the ocean
　　　　or in a park
I'd think about holding you.
　　　　　　reading stories to you.
　　　　　　and singing to you
I'd think about what it would.

be like to watch you grow,
I know I would have been
           proud of you
I could have loved you . . . I do
           love you now.

But I could have had you here
     to tell you that I love you . . .
looking at you or holding you
           close to me.
I could have loved you as a person
I knew, loved, and raised—
        not a person I just wonder
        about everyday
When you were still inside of me
and I thought these things,
           it was happy
because, for as long as I had you,
there was hope for days like those.
But that hope was taken away
     the day you were.
And when I think those things now,
I want to change what I did
because I miss you.

But missing you can't bring
     you back
     and tears can't bring you back.
I have to pay the consequences
        for my mistake,
           and the hardest part is
facing the fact that I can't get
     to know you now

You are and always will be
     my first child.
I think about you everyday
and I cry so many times.

I can't forget you
and I can't break the bond
between us
I don't want to
because you are very special
I didn't mean to hurt anyone
I really didn't.
Please help me to love
and to give
and to share
my gifts with others
like you would have
Help me to see the good
in others
Teach me to forgive those
who hurt me
as you forgive me for
hurting you
I'm sorry for taking away
your chance to share your gifts
God will take care of you
You're in His safe hands
I hope you are happy
I hope you aren't lonely without
the love of your parents
around you
I hope there are lots of kids
for you to play with
I hope you understand that
I do love you—although
I never got to see you here
I hope I will see you someday
and I hope you come to me
(smiling) when I reach out
my arms to you.

April 3, 1988

I cannot put flowers on your grave

I cannot put flowers on your grave,
for your funeral was a bucket or a bin
The only life I gave her,
Was death, borne of my sin.

You were born in the secret of darkness,
in the warmth and the love of my womb
And I killed you into security
as your harbor became your tomb.

You could hear my voice in your darkness,
You could hear my laugh or my cry.
But I, through ignorance could not,
Hear your pleas, not to die.

You loved me with trust and honesty
As you began your journey of life
I betrayed your innocence,
As I yielded to the Surgeon's knife.

The told me, I would be happier
That really it was all for the best.
I paid my money, succumbed to their lies,
And they tore you from my nest.

To abort you would solve my problems,
That's how they made their claims
Like lambs to the slaughter they led us,
And both of us, suffered such pain.

Forgive me dear child for my folly.
Of the horror I put you through.
Did you call out my name, "mummy,"
Just before I murdered you?

Your pain has long since been over,
Your death was your final release
But my life has been one of torment,
My heart pierced through with no peace.

Hear me, all mothers of the Universe,
Hear what I have to say.
Abortion is not the answer
It will not take your problems away.

For death is never the answer,
Take no heed to the vultures with knives
If you murder the life within you
You condemn not one, but two lives.

I cannot put flowers on your grave,
There's no marker to say that I care,
But in the barren desert of my heart,
A tiny rose blossoms there.

Anna was aborted on 24 September 1971.
Rest in peace my darling, in the arms of our God,
until I come home to you. —Mummy

25 September 1987

I wish there was something I could do or say.

I wish there was something I could do or say,
To turn back the hands of time,
And bring you, child, back to me.
I wish I could feel that flutter of life,
Just once more,
Before you are gone.
Some nights I want to hold you.
And know that you are safe and warm.
You never got a chance,
To feel the snow on your lashes,
The wind on your face,
Or the song of the dove in your heart.
I want you to know, my child, that I am very sorry,
That my life has become very sad,
And I miss you *very* much.